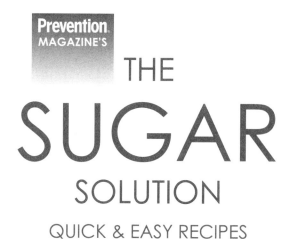

THE
SUGAR
SOLUTION
QUICK & EASY RECIPES

RODALE
LIVE YOUR WHOLE LIFE™

Every day our brands
connect with and inspire
millions of people to live
a life of the mind, body,
spirit — a whole life.

Prevention®
MAGAZINE'S

THE
SUGAR
SOLUTION
QUICK & EASY RECIPES

LOSE WEIGHT AND FEEL GREAT

Rosemary Ellis, editorial director, **Prevention®** magazine,
with Ann Fittante, MS, RD

RODALE

Portions of this book were previously published as Prevention's *The Sugar Solution Cookbook.*

© 2006 by Rodale Inc.

Photographs © 2006 by Rodale Inc.

Front cover recipe photographs are the Curried Tofu, page 150, and Peach and Raspberry Crostata, page 176.
Cover and recipe photographs by Mitch Mandel
Food styling by Diane Vezza
Book design by Christina Gaugler

Library of Congress Cataloging-in-Publication Data

Prevention magazine's the sugar solution quick & easy recipes : lose the weight and feel great / Rosemary Ellis, editorial director ; with Ann Fittante.
     p.   cm.
Includes index.
ISBN-13 978-1-59486-623-4 hardcover
ISBN-10 1-59486-623-6 hardcover
1. Sugar-free diet—Recipes. 2. Weight loss. I. Ellis, Rosemary. II. Fittante, Ann.
RM237.85P75 2006
641.5'638—dc22
                                               2006013286

2 4 6 8 10 9 7 5 3 1 hardcover

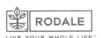

RODALE
LIVE YOUR WHOLE LIFE™

We inspire and enable people to improve their lives and the world around them
For more of our products visit **rodalestore.com** or call 800-848-4735

CONTENTS

THE SOLUTION
TO YOUR WEIGHT WOES

Heavenly pancakes studded with walnuts and slathered with rich maple-cream cheese. Savory Buffalo chicken bites served with creamy blue cheese. Soul-satisfying french fries. Peanut butter bundt cake. It sounds like a menu made in heaven. But in reality, these dishes—and many more—are part of a way of eating that can satisfy your tummy and slim your waistline. Without hunger. Without deprivation. And without food cravings that wake you out of a sound sleep at 2 a.m.

It's The Sugar Solution weight-loss program. This cookbook, full of quick and easy recipes, has more than 100 delicious dishes to help you bring the principles of this satisfying way of eating into your daily life. All the recipes are family friendly, and many are ready in less than 15 minutes, while many others can be prepared in 20 minutes or less.

And everyone in your family stands to benefit. The Sugar Solution is a safe and effective way of eating that can improve your body's ability to convert blood sugar—your body's primary source of energy—into fuel, rather than store it as fat. Ultimately, because the program prevents the dramatic surges and ebbs in blood sugar (also called glucose) that lead to food cravings, you're likely to find that you're satisfied with less food, and that your yen for sugary, fatty foods fades away.

In this book, you'll find all the information you need for experiencing the benefits of The Sugar Solution program for yourself.

- Get the latest news on the connection between blood sugar, insulin, and body weight.
- Learn why certain foods tend to blunt appetite and cravings—and why others keep you continuously ravenous.
- Discover how other lifestyle habits, like drinking enough water and getting plenty of sleep, can boost your weight loss efforts.

Best of all, The Sugar Solution will help you enjoy the foods you love while the pounds melt away. Page through the recipes in this cookbook and you'll find plenty of well-loved favorites—pasta, potatoes, bread, rice, and even cookies. That's right, you'll be enjoying carbohydrates. It's not necessary to banish carbs from your diet, if you choose the right ones in the right amounts. You'll find specific advice on finding the right carbs on page 2.

Ready to get started? Give *The Sugar Solution* a try and chances are, you'll be rewarded with a slimmer, healthier body—for good.

CHAPTER 1

THE SUGAR SOLUTION STRATEGY: A BEHIND-THE-SCENES GUIDE TO SUCCESSFUL WEIGHT LOSS

Ï f you're like many people, you've tried low-fat diets, high-protein diets, and the get-thin-quick diets found in popular magazines. But have they helped you lose weight and keep it off? In fact, if you're like most people who eventually quit them in frustration, you may have gained even *more* weight after following one of these diets.

Sound familiar? Don't beat yourself up. The problem may be in your blood—specifically, your blood sugar. Fortunately, so is the solution.

Let's begin with a rundown of what happens in the bloodstream when you eat. It's the first step toward understanding exactly how The Sugar Solution can help you lose weight.

It's in the Blood: The Science behind The Sugar Solution

Everyone has glucose in their blood. Glucose is the fuel that powers every cell in the body. When you eat, your body breaks down the food into glucose so it can enter the bloodstream. That process then triggers the pancreas to produce the hormone insulin. Think of insulin as a key that unlocks the cells, allowing glucose to enter. Once in the cells, glucose is either used for fuel or stored in the liver or muscles for future use.

How much insulin is needed to unlock cells depends on what we eat. Some foods take longer than others to break down into glucose. Those that break down slowly provide a lower amount of glucose for your body to absorb over a longer period of time; the pancreas responds by releasing insulin more slowly, too. Even better, when blood sugar rises gradually, it declines just as slowly over time. This gentle rise and fall actually discourages food cravings. However, when foods break down and enter the bloodstream quickly, the pancreas must quickly crank out a lot of insulin to ferry glucose from the blood into the cells. And once insulin has pushed glucose from the blood, glucose drops so low that it triggers cravings, overeating, and weight gain.

Essentially, the faster glucose enters the blood, the faster insulin rises—and the faster blood sugar plummets once that insulin begins to work. This pattern of rapid spikes and dips in your blood sugar level is a problem, both for your overall health and your weight.

Over time, the overeating that results can lead to excess body fat, which can cause cells to ignore insulin's signal to take glucose from the blood. In this condition (insulin resistance), glucose is locked out of the cells and converted to fat, which takes up even more real estate on the hips, waist, and behind.

Many advocates of low-carbohydrate weight-loss plans blame "carbohydrates" as the cause of our country's obesity epidemic. But in reality, no one gains weight by eating too many apples or too much oatmeal.

It's more accurate to say that different types of carbohydrates have different effects on blood sugar and the release of insulin. And those carbohydrates that cause the most dips and spikes in your blood sugar levels can leave you with terrible hunger pangs. Moreover, it's the excess calories consumed due to hunger-inducing fluctuations in blood sugar that cause weight gain.

Quick Carbs, Slow Carbs: How the Right Foods Can Help You Lose Weight

To better understand which foods are broken down into glucose more quickly than others, let's talk about carbohydrates. There are two basic categories of carbohydrates: unrefined and refined. Although they're both converted to glucose and raise blood sugar, they aren't converted at the same rate. How fast they're absorbed—and how much—is what impacts your weight.

Unrefined carbohydrates—found in plant foods like legumes, starchy vegetables, and whole grains—are rich in fiber and take longer to digest, which ultimately helps slow the body's absorption of the carbohydrates that these foods contain. Hence, these *slow carbs*, which delay the conversion of carbohydrates into glucose.

Refined carbohydrates—the kind in white bread, pasta, crackers, and baked goods—are a different story. Lacking the fiber that was removed when the grains were milled, these foods speed through the intestines and flood the bloodstream with glucose, causing insulin levels to zoom upward. Eat too many of these *quick carbs* and your body gets more glucose than it needs. That excess is turned into fat.

Even worse is that spike in insulin followed by a drop in blood sugar, which causes false "hunger" that is too often satisfied with even more quick carbs. It's a vicious cycle: You reach for quick carbs because you're hungry; your blood sugar and insulin skyrocket; then your blood sugar plunges leaving you blindsided by cravings, so you reach for more quick carbs because you're hungry—and your weight goes up, up, and away.

5 REASONS TO EAT THE SUGAR SOLUTION WAY

The healthy benefits of switching over to The Sugar Solution formula can be almost as dramatic as they are quick. Follow it faithfully, and here's what you can expect:

- Weight loss of $\frac{1}{2}$ pound to 2 pounds a week
- Fewer cravings for the sugary, fatty foods that cause weight gain
- More energy that lasts throughout the day
- Increased level of emotional well-being, self-confidence, and self-esteem
- Reduced risk of heart disease, diabetes, and cancer; researchers estimate that losing just 5 to 10 percent of body weight can reduce the risk of heart disease by lowering your blood pressure and cholesterol levels

It doesn't have to be this way. The Sugar Solution way of eating will wean you off the junk carbs at the root of your bottomless hunger. You'll learn how and what to eat to manage your blood sugar so you feel satisfied, not stuffed.

Lose Weight, Eat Great

The Sugar Solution way of eating is so satisfying that you'll never experience feelings of deprivation that can come with diets that restrict carbohydrates or fats. That's because this program is built around an irrefutable fact: Lasting weight loss isn't about eliminating *all* carbohydrates or avoiding every gram of fat that you find. It's about making smart choices.

On this program, you limit quick carbs and consume moderate amounts of slow carbs,

A SUPERCHARGED METABOLISM: JUST ADD WATER

Want to supercharge your calorie-burning potential? Drink up, says Ann Fittante, MS, RD. It seems that fluids—especially plain water—really can support weight-loss efforts. Researchers in Germany measured the resting metabolism of 14 men and women before and after they drank just over 16 ounces of water. Within 10 minutes, their metabolisms began to rise, and after 40 minutes, their average calorie-burning rate was 30 percent higher. And it stayed elevated for more than an hour.

Researchers don't understand why, but they calculate that drinking eight cups (64 ounces) of water a day—the generally recommended amount—can burn off almost 35,000 calories a year, or about 10 pounds.

But you don't need to drown in the stuff. A recent National Academy of Sciences report found that most women need 11 cups (88 ounces) of fluid a day, but it doesn't all have to be water. A cup of tea counts, as does juice or the occasional diet cola. (Limit or eliminate sugary sodas and juices, though. Studies show that liquid calories don't register on your hunger radar and can sneak up on your waistline.) It's safe to drink a total of 8 to 12 cups a day. And drink it cool—part of the increased calorie burn occurs as the body warms the liquid to body temperature.

Sweet Success
BETH SHAW

Thirty-eight-year-old yoga instructor Beth Shaw was skinny as a rail until she turned 16. "I had a sedentary after-school job, and a good part of my income went to burgers, Chinese food, and pizza," says the resident of Hermosa Beach, California. In a matter of months, Beth had gained 25 pounds.

With diet and exercise, the 5-foot-11 woman shed those pounds—and more—and stayed slender for a few years. "In college, I weighed 135 pounds. I was borderline anorexic," she says. Eventually, however, the scale headed north once again.

Beth was at her highest weight—185 pounds—in 1989, when she moved from her native New York City to Los Angeles. Alone in an unfamiliar place, toiling at a stressful job, food was her consolation. "I sat from 6:45 a.m. to 5 p.m. but was constantly tired and stressed," she says. "I felt fat, helpless, and depressed. My weight—and my life—were out of control."

Determined to ease her stress, Beth began to practice yoga. Something clicked. "It put me in touch with my body, reduced my stress, and improved my mood." She began to study yoga and in 1993 began to teach it. Shortly thereafter, she created YogaFit, a hybrid style of yoga that emphasizes fitness.

But though her business was a smashing success, Beth was still battling her extra pounds. Her weight seesawed until 1995 when she met a personal trainer at one of her yoga retreats. On his advice, the 175-pound Beth began an eating plan that emphasized low-glycemic carbohydrates.

Breakfast was two eggs with oatmeal or a protein drink. At midmorning, she nibbled on a low-carb snack bar. Lunch was sushi or a green salad with tuna or chicken. In the midafternoon, Beth snacked on a piece of fruit with a handful of nuts or a protein drink. For dinner, she enjoyed fish, chicken, or steak; a salad; and a small sweet potato. Beth also lifted weights and did cardio along with her yoga.

"My weight began to drop instantly," she says. A year later, she was 20 pounds lighter.

Beth now weighs between 150 and 153 pounds and wears a size 6–8. She lifts weights twice a week, walks with her dogs, and practices some form of yoga 5 days a week. Last fall, she ran a half-marathon. "I feel calm and in control," she says.

lean proteins, and healthy fats. You'll also practice portion control and eat smaller, more frequent meals. All of these strategies help the insulin "key" efficiently go about its business of unlocking cells, leaving little surplus glucose hanging around to be stored as fat. As a bonus, normalizing glucose and insulin levels tend to boost energy. You'll have more incentive to work out regularly and be less inclined to reach for sweets at midafternoon.

The Sugar Solution recipes are based on the glycemic index (GI), which ranks foods based on how swiftly and how much they raise blood sugar. Foods with a low GI—typically healthy, slow carbs—are converted to glucose more slowly than those with a medium or high GI (typically quick carbs). Eating lower on the GI scale benefits insulin and blood sugar levels, which in turn discourages fat storage. And because fiber-rich, low-GI foods stay in your system longer, they keep you full and discourage the overeating that leads to weight gain. The recipes in this cookbook are prepared with lower-GI ingredients such as beans, grains, and whole grain flours and pastas.

SLEEP MORE, LOSE MORE

If you sleep less than 8 hours a night, getting more Zs may help you lose weight. Sleep deprivation disrupts your body's normal ability to process and control various weight-related hormones, including glucose and cortisol. This imbalance encourages cells to store excess fat, lowers your body's fat-burning ability, and may make it tougher to control cravings.

But just 9 hours of sleep for 3 consecutive nights can reverse this, making weight loss easier. Here's a trio of sleepy-time tips.

Take a brisk, after-dinner walk. Regular exercise—30 minutes most days of the week—reduces stress and raises body temperature, which primes you for slumber.

Each evening, prep for sleep. Take a bath, listen to relaxing music, and make sure your bedroom is dark, cool, and quiet.

Nap to nip cravings. If you've endured a sleepless night, take a 10-minute nap the next day. It will improve both your mood and your ability to stick to your diet.

THE SUGAR SOLUTION SAFETY FEATURES

Ever struggled through a low-carb diet and shed your hair along with the pounds? Or felt like death warmed over on one of those 800-calorie-a-day fad diets? Unlike nutritionally unbalanced, overly stringent weight-loss plans, The Sugar Solution program was designed with your health and satisfaction in mind. Here's why:

- **It's not a fad.** The Sugar Solution plan is based on the current recommendations in medical and nutritional literature. It doesn't exclude major food groups (hint: carbohydrates) or advocate pricey supplements.

- **It's nutritionally sound.** You get the nutrients you need for energy and good health—not the case with many low-carb or low-calorie diets. Each meal is packed with vitamins, minerals, fiber, and health-promoting plant compounds from a balanced mix of complex carbohydrates, lean proteins, and good fats.

- **It contains enough calories.** You'll consume between 1,400 and 1,600 calories a day. This range is low enough to promote safe weight loss but not low enough to slow your metabolism or cause you to feel ill or exhausted.

- **It won't lead to hair loss.** Some women on low-carb plans complain of losing their hair along with their excess pounds, perhaps because these diets skimp on nutrients. With this program, your hair stays on your head.

- **It won't cause gallstones.** Very low calorie diets of 800 calories or less are associated with gallstones. These solid chunks of material form in the gallbladder—the pear-shaped organ that produces bile, which aids in digestion—and can get stuck in the gallbladder duct, causing pain and infection. (It's thought that rapid weight loss reduces the gallbladder's ability to contract and send bile into the intestine.) On The Sugar Solution plan, weight loss is slow, which reduces the risk of gallstones.

- **It's safe for people with diabetes.** Low-carb diets can cause ketosis, in which the body burns fat for fuel instead of carbohydrates. Ketosis is dangerous for some people with diabetes. On this plan, you never go into ketosis, because at least half your diet is carbohydrates. (However, people with diabetes who follow *any* weight-loss plan should step up their blood-glucose monitoring and contact their doctor if they experience low blood sugar.)

CHAPTER 2

THE SUGAR SOLUTION PLAN: 4 SIMPLE PRINCIPLES (AND 16 EASY TIPS) FOR SUCCESS

Now that you understand the science behind The Sugar Solution program, it's time to put the plan into practice. Follow the 16 basic steps, and you're off to a great start. Focus on one a day, if that's easier for you. Simply live and cook by the four simple principles below and the weight will melt away, along with your food cravings and fatigue.

Principle 1: Upgrade Your Carbs

Craving a juicy McIntosh apple or a warm and crunchy slice of whole grain toast? Enjoy. On The Sugar Solution program, you don't eliminate carbohydrates, you upgrade them—that is, trade in the quick carbs that encourage weight gain for the slow carbs that dampen your appetite and discourage excess body fat. Live by this principle, watch your portion sizes, and you'll find it's easier not only to lose weight but to keep it off. You'll also eat hearty with none of the deprivation of most low-carb menu plans, and your body will get the vitamins, minerals, and other substances essential to good health.

As you'll see, we've upgraded the carbohydrates in our recipes with mouthwatering results. Our Carrot Cake Pancakes (page 44) are made with whole grain pastry flour. The Spicy Corn and Sweet Potato Chowder (page 58) lends an old-fashioned favorite—traditionally made with white potatoes—a new and tasty twist. Love chocolate pudding? Turn to page 179 to see how we've made a good thing even better with low-fat, low-glycemic ingredients.

Upgrading your carbs is simpler than you think. Here are four easy ways to do it. As you'll see, sometimes the glycemic index (GI) of a particular food matters less than its content of vitamins, minerals, and health-protective plant chemicals.

- Upgrade from white to sweet potatoes. Of course, you can eat a small spud every now and again. But there are good reasons to make the moist, orange-fleshed spud a regular indulgence. Not only is the GI of a sweet potato much lower than that of a regular potato (54 versus 85), but sweet potatoes are packed with beta-carotene, vitamins C and E, and fiber. Try a small, baked sweet potato, sprinkled with cinnamon and artificial sweetener. Or bake up some sweet potato fries. Preheat the oven to 450°F. Coat a baking sheet with cooking spray. Slice 2 medium sweet potatoes or yams (peels on, for extra fiber) into ½"-thick wedges. Combine the potatoes, 1 tablespoon of olive oil, ¼ teaspoon of salt, and ⅛ teaspoon of pepper in a bowl and toss well. Arrange the potatoes in a single layer on the baking sheet. Bake for 30 to 45 minutes, turning halfway through. Serve immediately.

- Upgrade from white to whole grain pastas. Their GI is nearly identical (41 for white spaghetti, 37 for whole wheat). However, the latter contains more fiber and healthy plant nutrients than the former. They pack more flavor, too—many people come to love the chewy, nutty-tasting whole wheat pastas. If you don't, Eden Foods offers a hybrid pasta that combines 60 percent whole grain flour with refined flour. You'll find it in natural food stores or in some large supermarkets, or visit www.edenfoods.com. And check the stores for other whole grain pastas made with brown rice, corn, spelt, and buckwheat.

- Upgrade from white to whole grain bread. Again, both varieties of bread are similar on the GI scale, because when fiber is finely ground, as it often is in whole wheat flour, it doesn't present enough of a digestive challenge to lower the GI of foods made with it. However, whole wheat bread is a healthier choice because of its extra fiber and other nutrients. Best bets include Pepperidge Farm 100% Stone Ground Whole Wheat Bread, Wonder Stone Ground 100% Whole Wheat Bread, and Thomas' Sahara 100% Whole Wheat Pita Bread. Tried 'em and don't like 'em—or can't get used to 'em? When you make a sandwich, do some sleight of hand: Put a slice of your favorite bread on top, and use whole grain bread on the bottom. Or use whole grain bread to make your own bread crumbs.

Discover one new whole grain a month. From amaranth to wild rice, there's a dazzling array of whole grains from around the world to bring to your table. For example, cooked quinoa (pronounced KEEN-wa) is excellent in casseroles, soups, stews, and stir-fries (and cooks in about 15 minutes). You can even cook it in fruit juice and enjoy it as a breakfast cereal, or use it cold in salads. And bulgur is delicious as a side dish that doesn't require stove-top cooking. Your local natural food store will have 'em all. To field-test these great grains, try our delicious Curried Couscous Salad (page 83), Quinoa with Raisins, Apricots, and Pecans (page 106), and Mediterranean Couscous (page 109).

Principle 2: Eat Less, More Often

Mom probably told you to eat three square meals a day, but that may be bad advice when you're trying to lose weight. Research has found that women who eat large meals may burn 60 fewer calories per day than those who eat smaller amounts of food every few hours. And while 60 calories a day may not sound like much, it's the equivalent of 6 pounds a year.

On The Sugar Solution program, you eat small amounts more frequently—every 3 hours or so. These mini-meals can keep your blood sugar on an even keel, which dampens food cravings and prevents the spikes in insulin that promote fat storage. And there's plenty of compelling evidence that this eat-less-more-often strategy works. Researchers at the University of Massachusetts in Worcester found that people who eat four or more times daily—generally three meals and one or two snacks—are less likely to be obese than those who eat fewer meals.

Eating every few hours may seem an unlikely way to save calories, if you usually skip meals or starve yourself to lose weight—until you consider that these methods actually slow your metabolism. It's true. When you starve yourself, the body senses that food is scarce and conserves its reserves, slowing its metabolism to hold on to what it has until the next big meal comes along.

For success on The Sugar Solution plan, follow these mini-meal do's and don'ts.

TEAM YOUR WILLPOWER WITH SKILLPOWER

When it comes to weight loss, you need more than willpower. You need skillpower—the ability to solve problems and strategize when things get tough and your resolution to be good evaporates. Willpower is like a car's engine: It gets you revved up to go. But skillpower is the steering wheel that helps you navigate obstacles. These tips can help you hone this expertise.

Set smaller, more doable goals. In the beginning, willpower is strong and intoxicating. You think you'll do everything perfectly—no more sweets, an hour-long workout a day, skimpy portions—and by summer, you'll look like a *Sports Illustrated* swimsuit model. Skillpower says forget the bikini and focus on fitting into last year's shorts. Rewarding yourself for achieving small goals like this keeps skillpower sharp and motivation high.

Plan ahead to avoid danger zones. Hanging out with friends at a coffeehouse while your mouth waters over the chocolate croissants requires iron willpower. The smarter skillpower way: Get your coffee to go and chat while you take a brisk, croissant-free walk together.

Catch yourself quickly. If you raid the office vending machine at 4 p.m., you're likely to hit the cookies when you arrive home from the office. Use skillpower to get back on track and eat a healthy dinner. A Brown University study of 142 people reports that if you get back on the diet-and-exercise track immediately after a binge, your weight loss efforts won't suffer.

Avoid portion distortion. The idea is to feed your body enough to keep your hunger at bay and your metabolism revving. If you overfuel, you defeat the whole purpose of eating small. To make sure your mini-meals are truly mini, use a salad plate as a dinner plate and a coffee cup as a bowl. As you'll see, the meals in this book are rarely more than 600 calories, and snacks top out at 150 calories.

Follow the formula. Each mini-meal should contain a balance of nutrients, including slow carbs, protein, and healthy fat. Don't worry about looking up nutrition guidelines to calculate the exact ratios—just make sure that all three nutrients are included in what you select. For example, a healthy mini might be half a turkey sandwich (no cheese) on whole grain bread with ½ teaspoon of light mayo and a piece of fruit; or a mini-pita with 1 tablespoon of hummus and 5 baby carrots.

Start your day with a mini-meal. Studies show that breakfast eaters tend to lose more weight when dieting than do breakfast skippers. But that's not a green light to order the Farmer's Breakfast Special at the diner every morning. Instead, apply the mini-meal formula here, too. You might scramble two egg whites with spinach and wrap it in a small whole grain tortilla, or enjoy ½ cup of oatmeal with half an orange and a cheese stick.

Choose maxi-nutrient minis. Don't be tempted by the small packages that lurk in the snack aisle or inside vending machines. A tiny bag of chips or half a candy bar might look mini, but you'll be cheating yourself out of nutrients—and put yourself right back on that blood sugar roller coaster. Ditto for the new snack products that tout only 100 calories per serving. It's not always calories that count: You'll need to weigh your selections by the amount of quick carbs they contain as well.

Principle 3: Eat One Bowl of High-Fiber Cereal a Day

Cereal lovers, rejoice! Not only does The Sugar Solution allow this breakfast favorite on the menu, it encourages you to enjoy it. That's because eating just 1 serving a day can provide as much as 15 grams of fiber—half, or more than half, of the 25 to 30 grams experts recommend.

Of course, adding more fiber to your diet is a healthy choice. But it's also a smart move if you're looking to drop some weight. In a 2003 study, researchers at the Harvard School of Public Health linked diets high in whole grains to lowered weight gain.

Over a 12-year period, the researchers followed the eating habits of more than 74,000 women to study the association between whole grain intake and weight gain over time. What they found: The more whole grains the women consumed, the less they tended to weigh. Moreover, women who ate the most fiber had a 49 percent lower risk of weight gain than women who consumed the lowest amount of fiber. It may be that whole grains promote weight loss because they give that tummy-satisfying feeling of fullness (researchers call it satiety) or because they influence the body's use of insulin.

If you plan to follow our makeover, feel free to swap any of the suggested snacks for your bowl-a-day. You can also opt to have cereal for breakfast as many times a week as you wish. And try these tips.

Spoon up the right portion. Successful weight loss begins with correct portion sizes. Eat 1 serving of cereal for breakfast, $\frac{1}{2}$ serving for a snack (with $\frac{1}{2}$ cup of fat-free or soymilk). Use a measuring cup for a week until you're certain you know what 1 serving really looks like.

Make your cereal berry sweet. Give your cereal an extra blast of flavor as well as fiber,

---

THE SUGAR SOLUTION CEREAL SAFARI

Finding a whole grain cereal got easier in 2004, when General Mills announced that it would make all its cereals with whole grains. Opt for a brand that contains at least 7 grams of fiber. The cereals that follow are low in calories and sugar and are good sources of appetite-blunting slow carbs.

- All-Bran with Extra Fiber (1 cup) 100 calories, 15 grams fiber
- Fiber One ($\frac{1}{2}$ cup) 118 calories, 14 grams fiber
- Kashi Seven Whole Grains & Sesame ($\frac{3}{4}$ cup) 90 calories, 8 grams fiber
- General Mills Multi-Bran Chex (1 cup) 200 calories, 8 grams fiber

Sweet Success

CARSON REDWINE

Carson Redwine, a welfare worker in Muncie, Indiana, started to gain weight after his 30th birthday. "I was less active than I used to be and didn't change my eating habits," says Carson, now 53. As he continued to gain, he tried to cut back on doughnuts, bread, chips, and cookies. Unfortunately, he failed. By 2000, Carson carried almost 300 pounds on his 6-foot-1 frame.

"I knew I had a problem," he says. "I woke up at night short of breath. Taking my daily walk with my wife, Anna, was becoming more difficult. When I bent over to tie my shoelaces, it was hard to breathe. My weight made me self-conscious, and I was upset with myself for allowing myself to get so heavy." He vowed to lose weight for good.

In March 2003, he turned his eating habits around, abandoning the quick carbs that contributed to his weight gain and low energy levels. "At first, I was miserable," says Carson. But it wasn't long before he started to feel better, physically and mentally.

Carson started his day with slow carbs: a cup of oatmeal topped with a handful of walnuts or pecans or slices of fresh fruit. Sometimes, he enjoyed two organic eggs prepared with olive oil and his own homemade, fiber-full whole wheat toast. Lunch was a piece of fruit, a slice of cheese, a slice of his bread spread with peanut butter, and a glass of milk, or a bowl of his homemade bean or chicken-vegetable soup. For dinner, he enjoyed broiled or baked fish or chicken, a baked sweet potato, salad, and a green vegetable. Between meals, Carson snacked on nuts and fruit and drank plenty of water and green tea.

Over a 20-month period, Carson lost almost 50 pounds, and he now weighs 247 pounds. He'd like to get down to 170 pounds—his weight when he got married at age 19—and is "actively pursuing that goal."

Carson has continued his daily walks, which have become much easier. "Anna and I walk 2 to 3 miles a day," he says. "We also do Leslie Sansone's Walk Away the Pounds. Her workouts are excellent for people of all ages."

Carson says that his life has changed for the better. "I no longer doze off when I sit down," he says. "I sleep better. I'm more active. And I'm in control, not the potato chips and soft drinks. Now I think about what I eat."

with berries. Just ½ cup of fresh raspberries contains 4 grams of fiber; ½ cup of frozen blue-berries has 2 grams of fiber. (Feel free to use a sugar substitute as well.)

Splash on the soy. Both regular and vanilla low-fat soymilk are a delicious twist on reg-ular skim milk and a good option if you're lactose intolerant or allergic to cow's milk. Look for calcium-fortified brands with calcium and vitamin D at about the same levels as dairy milk: 300 milligrams of calcium, 100 IU of vitamin D per 8 ounces. A few to try: Silk Vanilla, 8th Continent Vanilla, or WestSoy Plus Vanilla.

Sprinkle on the flax. Mixing 1 tablespoon of high-fiber, ground flaxseed into your cereal can help curb your appetite and eliminate calories. Flaxseed is also a rich source of alpha-linoleic acid (ALA), an important omega-3 fat that protects against high cholesterol, diabetes, and high blood pressure. You'll find flaxseed at health food stores or natural food supermarkets. Refrigerate promptly since the delicate oil in flaxseed can go rancid easily.

Principle 4: Don't Skimp on Good Fats

If you've tried the popular high-protein diets, you're probably sick of the sight of bacon, steak, and pork rinds. That's good, because much of the fat on these plans is derived from the unhealthy saturated fats found in butter, fatty red meats, and full-fat dairy products. Many quick carbs—cookies, cakes, and crackers—tend to contain trans fats, which are just as unhealthy as saturated fats, if not more so. Trans fats—created when hydrogen gas reacts with oil—raise bad LDL cholesterol, like saturated fats do, but also crush heart-protective HDL cholesterol. Further, these "frankenfats" have been linked to cancer and diabetes.

However, a diet stripped of fat isn't healthy, either. Your body needs fat to function prop-erly. Dietary fat also stabilizes blood sugar levels, which helps you feel full and satisfied for hours.

On The Sugar Solution program, you'll consume from 25 to 30 percent of your total daily calories from fat, most of that derived from healthy fats such as olive oil, natural peanut butter and other nut butters, and avocados. Cold-water fish such as salmon, walnuts, almonds, flaxseed, and canola oil contain heart-healthy omega-3 fatty acids.

As you'll see in the recipes, we swap butter for olive oil, forgo full-fat cheese and sour cream for the reduced-fat kind, and use the leanest cuts of beef and pork. So go ahead, dig into the Grilled Peppered Steak with Multigrain Texas Toast (page 113). You'll consume just 5 grams of fat per serving.

If you're following the 28-day program, we've calculated your fat budget for you. Once you're on your own, however, there are simple ways to make sure you choose good fats over bad. Trade your grilled steak or burger for grilled salmon once a week, and ditch the bacon bits on your salads and top them with nuts or seeds for a flavorful crunch.

Keep the following tips in mind and you'll be sure to get the good fats you need.

Eat a good-fat appetizer to crush cravings. Marshall Goldberg, MD, an endocrinologist at Thomas Jefferson University Medical College in Philadelphia, found that spreading 2 teaspoons of olive oil on half a slice of bread eaten 15 to 20 minutes before a meal helps his patients control their cravings. Olive oil is known to stimulate the release of cholecystokinin (CCK), a gut hormone that signals the brain to stop eating. It may be that olive oil also slows stomach contractions, which creates a sense of fullness. (Of course, make your bread whole grain.)

Feast on fatty fish twice a week. Salmon is an easy way to get your omega-3s, called eicosapentaenoic acid (EPA) and docosahexaenoic acid (DHA). A serving of salmon the size of a deck of cards (about 3 ounces) will bring you almost 2 grams of EPA and DHA. Or have a tuna salad sandwich. Buy canned white albacore tuna in water (light tuna has less omega-3s). Use low-fat mayo or mayo made from canola oil.

Go nuts. Sprinkle 2 tablespoons of toasted, chopped nuts a day on your whole grain cereal, low-fat yogurt, salads, or stir-fries. And feel free to indulge in 1 serving (2 tablespoons) of all-natural peanut butter, which doesn't contain trans fats or added sugar.

Switch to trans free margarines. A few to try: Land O Lakes Light Country Morning Blend, I Can't Believe It's Not Butter with Yogurt!, Promise Ultra Spread, and Spectrum Naturals Spread (sold in natural food stores).

Sweet Success

MARY KONIZ ARNOLD

Mary Koniz Arnold, 43, gained weight after getting married and having kids. "My food choices changed. I went from choosing skinless chicken to bratwurst, brown rice to biscuits," she says. Her stressful job at a nonprofit agency included food at every special event and meeting.

Mary felt fit and stayed active—"I walked or jogged every day, swam at the Y, rode my bike, and danced." But by 2000, the 5-foot-1 Mary weighed 217 pounds. Around that time, she bought a pair of size 20 pants and felt compelled to buy a girdle for her 20-year high-school reunion.

The weight began to come off when Mary made modest changes in her diet and started teaching gymnastics part-time. "I took my daughter to her class one day, and they were short-staffed," she says. "I had done gymnastics as a child, and I could still do the moves, so I offered to help."

Her first year teaching gymnastics, she lost 10 pounds. Changing jobs in 2002—Mary is now a writer/photographer at a community college in Poughkeepsie, New York—helped her lose another 10. "I walked more and had less access to food," she says.

Mary kept off those 20 pounds and even completed a half-marathon in 2003. In the spring of 2004, before training for a full marathon, she developed a knee problem. An orthopedist recommended physical therapy—and weight loss. "Exercise wasn't enough anymore. I had to change my diet drastically," she says. She was at 197 pounds.

She joined a weight-loss program offering support meetings and guidance in food choices. A typical breakfast: oatmeal with fruit, ½ cup of fat-free milk, and ⅓ cup of fat-free cottage cheese. Lunch was brown rice and beans with salsa and fat-free cheese, or lean meat and a salad. Dinner: 2 ounces of lean meat, 1 cup of whole grain pasta or brown rice, salad, and cooked vegetables. Snacks included fruit, fat-free cheese, raw veggies, and whole grain cereal with fruit and skim milk.

In 8 months, she lost another 60 pounds and now weighs 137 pounds. "Yesterday I bought a pair of pants—size 2!" she says.

She's running again, and dropping 80 pounds has allowed her to surpass her childhood gymnastics skills. "I always loved the balance beam, but now I do the uneven bars, too—pullovers, back hip circles, mill circles, and jumping to the high bar," she says. "I'm still working on my back handspring."

CHAPTER 3

STOCKING THE SUGAR SOLUTION KITCHEN

The Sugar Solution lifestyle doesn't just transform your body, it transforms your kitchen. Since you'll be spending less time at the drive-through window and more time preparing your own healthy, tasty meals, there's a good chance that your pantry, refrigerator, and freezer need a drastic overhaul. Fortunately, our Kitchen Makeover—which takes just minutes—will make losing extra pounds and adopting healthier eating habits much easier.

The biggest benefit? Having the right foods on hand prevents slips and binges that can slow your weight loss or derail your efforts altogether. When you don't keep quick carbs and bad fats in your house, they can't undermine your good intentions. Similarly, if you stock your kitchen with slow carbs and good fats, you won't break into your husband's chips or your children's lunchbox snacks because there's nothing else to eat.

What's more, cooking and eating at home takes much less time than you think. You might spend 5 minutes planning your weekly menu, 30 minutes a week at the supermarket, and 20 minutes a day in the kitchen preparing dinner (less for breakfast and lunch). When you think about it, preparing healthy meals takes about as much time as sitting in your car at the drive-through or waiting in line at the local takeout place.

This chapter is a guide to stocking your kitchen with Sugar Solution–friendly foods.

When you shop smart, you put the makings for fresh, healthy meals right where you need them: in your pantry, refrigerator, and freezer. Follow our easy three-step Kitchen Makeover and you'll be able to whip up meals that please your tastebuds (and your waistline) in less time than it takes the pizza guy to ring your doorbell.

Step 1: Put Your Kitchen on a Diet

In this step, you ferret out the quick carbs and bad fats lurking in your pantry, refrigerator, and freezer. Toss the following waist-thickening foods, or box up unopened items and donate them to charity.

- Boxed dinner mixes or high-fat, high-calorie frozen dinners
- Bread, bagels, or English muffins that are not whole grain
- Frozen convenience foods, such as french fries and fish sticks
- Full-fat ice cream
- Full-sugar jellies and jams
- High-fat lunchmeats (salami, bologna, pepperoni)
- High-fat meats
- High-fat processed meats, such as bacon, sausage, and hot dogs
- Most canned soups, stews, and pasta meals
- Most salad dressings (unless they're free of trans fats)
- Packaged cookies, baked goods, and other sweets
- Pasta and noodles made from white flour
- Processed cheese in cans
- Salty snack foods
- Stick margarine (unless it's free of trans fats)
- Sugar-coated cereals, or those that are not whole grain
- Sugar-sweetened yogurt
- Sugary soft drinks and juices

Step 2: Restock with Healthy Foods

When you've completed Step 1, you should be left with mostly slow carbs and good fats. These foods include:

- All-natural peanut butter or other nut butter
- Eggs
- Fresh or frozen fish, such as tuna, sardines, or salmon, or canned tuna and salmon in water
- Fresh or frozen fruits and vegetables
- Frozen juice bars with no sugar added
- Lean meats and poultry (chicken, turkey breast, or very lean ground beef)
- Low-fat bottled marinara sauce
- Low-fat dairy or soy products
- Nuts prepared without salt or fat (raw almonds, walnuts, no-salt peanuts)
- Olive, flax, and canola oils
- Whole grain breads, cereals, and pastas

Step 3: Go Forth and Shop!

You say your cupboards (and fridge and freezer) are bare? It's time to restock them with healthy fare. Below you'll find lists of foods to fill them with, by category, along with some tasty cooking tips. No need to buy every item listed: Let your personal tastes guide your selections. But do be adventurous and buy items you've never tried before.

FRUITS AND VEGETABLES

Buy these:

- Canned or frozen legumes
- Canned vegetables (optional; buy low-sodium, or drain and rinse before use)

- Edamame (Japanese whole soybeans)
- Fresh fruit (apples, bananas, blueberries, exotic fruits, grapefruit, grapes, melon, oranges, strawberries)
- Fresh herbs (basil, cilantro, parsley, rosemary, tarragon, and thyme)
- Fresh vegetables (broccoli, cabbage, carrots, celery, collard greens, cucumber, green/red/yellow peppers, kale, mushrooms, onions, squash, tomatoes, zucchini)
- Frozen berries
- Frozen vegetables prepared without fat or fatty sauces
- Packaged greens (including spinach) for salads
- Scallions (green onions)
- Sweet potatoes
- Winter squash

Tasty tips:

- Because frozen veggies are frozen at the peak of ripeness, they're often more nutritious than the fresh stuff that's been languishing in the produce bins. Go for Asian stir-fry or other mixes that include one or more of the following: broccoli, carrots, cauliflower, and Brussels sprouts.
- Tuck veggies in every sandwich—and not just a token lettuce leaf. Pick up prewashed bagged greens with big flavor power, such as baby spinach, arugula, and mesclun mix. Or try precut coleslaw mix (shredded cabbage and carrots).
- Kale, mustard and turnip greens, and Swiss chard are delicious, chock-full of healthy phytochemicals, and easy to prepare. Just wash, cut off the tough bottom stems, and sauté until limp in olive oil seasoned with garlic, ginger, or other spices.
- Fresh herbs and scallions add zip and flavor to many foods. Snip and top on salads.
- Crushed, peeled tomatoes or plain diced tomatoes in juice can be used in a wide variety of dishes. No-added-salt tomato sauce can be used on pizza or mixed with a commercial pasta sauce to lower its sodium content.

- Like veggies, fruits are flash-frozen at their ripest. Your best-tasting and most nutritious bets: berries (loaded with antioxidants) and mangoes (with beta-carotene). Toss ½ cup each of blueberries and raspberries into a smoothie, or add to pancakes and breads.
- Edamame is available at most natural food stores either fresh or frozen. Cook in the pod and serve as an appetizer.
- Cut sweet potatoes lengthwise into eight wedges per potato. Place in a bowl and toss with a little olive oil and paprika. Spread on a baking sheet that has been coated with nonstick spray and bake in a 450°F oven, turning once, for 30 to 45 minutes, until golden brown.
- Stir unsweetened applesauce or a little curry powder into cooked, solid-pack frozen squash and serve as a side dish.

WHOLE GRAIN BREADS, CEREALS, AND PASTAS

Buy these:

- Barley
- Brown rice
- Bulgur
- High-fiber/low-sugar hot and cold cereal
- Oatmeal (whole oats) or steel-cut oats
- Whole grain bread and English muffins
- Whole wheat couscous
- Whole wheat or corn tortillas
- Whole wheat or whole grain pasta

Tasty tips:

- Heat small whole wheat or corn tortillas briefly in a skillet, then roll with a combination of diced cooked chicken, cooked pinto beans or black beans, diced scallion, roasted red pepper, and a bit of cheese. Heat until the cheese melts.
- To make a crispy snack, brush 1 whole wheat tortilla with a teaspoon of olive oil, and sprinkle with your favorite seasonings (chili powder, garlic, salt, pepper). Cut into 12 wedges. Arrange on a lightly oiled baking sheet. Bake at 350°F for 5 to 10 minutes, until crisp. Cool on paper towels and enjoy. Makes 1 serving.

- Couscous is a form of pasta usually made from refined wheat flour. Use the whole wheat kind (available in natural food supermarkets), and you'll score 7 grams of craving-busting fiber per serving, compared with just 2 grams in regular couscous.
- Toasting barley gives it a light, nutty flavor. Place the barley in a nonstick skillet over medium heat. Cook, stirring or shaking constantly, for 5 minutes, or until grain is golden.
- Bake brown rice! Combine rice and liquid (chicken, beef, or vegetable broth) in a casserole dish. Cover and bake at 375°F for 25 minutes, or until the liquid is absorbed.

LOW-FAT DAIRY PRODUCTS

Buy these:

- Fat-free milk or soymilk
- Fat-free or low-fat cottage cheese
- Fat-free or low-fat yogurt (plain or flavored)
- Reduced-fat cheese (as well as lower fat cheeses like goat cheese and part-skim mozzarella)
- Small amount of highly flavored cheese, such as Parmesan, Blue cheese, or Cheddar (used as a condiment)

Tasty tips:

- Reduced-fat cheese has come a long way—the quality and taste are better than ever. Try low-fat cheese on whole grain crackers and sandwiches, or shred some over your veggies at dinner.
- A number of cheeses, such as aged sharp Cheddar, feta, and grated Parmesan or Romano, add a lot of flavor in small amounts. Use as you would a condiment—approximately 1 tablespoon to flavor eggs, pasta, or salads.
- Use fat-free or low-fat plain yogurt as a lower-fat, higher-calcium stand-in for sour cream or mayonnaise.
- Don't use a lot of yogurt? Buy an 8-ounce container and replace as needed.

Sweet Success
FRAN EHRET

On Valentine's Day 2002, Fran Ehret, then 60, received a sugary surprise. But it wasn't a heart-shaped box of chocolates. It was a diabetes diagnosis from his doctor.

The retired postmaster from Hellertown, Pennsylvania, was told that his blood sugar was a staggering 190 mg/dl. (Diabetes is diagnosed at 126 mg/dl.) Moreover, at 5 feet 8 inches and 200 pounds, Fran was obese. If he didn't lose weight, his doctor said, he'd have to take insulin.

"That scared me," says Fran, now 62. His brother, a diabetic, had passed away at 62. His father, also a diabetic, had died of a heart attack at 63.

"I was a time bomb waiting to happen," says Fran. "I used to not care about what I ate or when I ate it." His biggest weakness was eating at night. His cravings typically started right after dinner, when he snacked on potato chips, sausage, or bologna and cheese, and ended only when he nodded off in front of the TV.

"I wasn't ready to die," Fran says. Determined to take charge of his health, he overhauled his eating habits.

Instead of the quick carbs he usually ate for breakfast—doughnuts and sugar-laden coffee, or a cheesesteak omelet, home fries, and white toast slathered with butter—he had a bowl of whole grain cereal with 1 percent milk and a cup of tea. Lunch was tuna salad (made with low-fat salad dressing) on whole wheat bread rather than a sandwich piled high with lunchmeat. For dinner, Fran switched from red meat, mashed potatoes, and white bread to fish, chicken, or whole wheat pasta and two vegetables prepared without fat.

As Fran trimmed his diet, he ramped up his activity levels. He began to walk an hour a day, either outdoors or on his treadmill, which he moved from the basement into the sunroom so that he could use it while watching TV.

In just a few months, Fran shed 30 pounds. Napping during the day or nodding off in front of the TV was a thing of the past. "My energy levels were through the roof," he says. Three years later, Fran has kept off every last pound, continues to stick to his healthy diet and daily walks, and still has energy to burn. "And the last time my doctor checked my blood sugar, it was normal," says Fran. "No insulin for me."

LEGUMES

Buy these:

- All varieties of beans—garbanzo, pinto, white, navy, black
- Lentils

Tasty tips:

- Some supermarkets carry legumes, such as black beans or pinto beans, in the frozen foods section. If you find them, snap them up. Frozen legumes are lower in sodium and have a firmer texture than canned beans. Also, you can add small amounts of frozen beans to your dishes without wondering what to do with the rest of the can.

---

5 SMART WAYS TO DO SOY

Slash waist-thickening (and artery-clogging) saturated fat with these great-tasting soy versions of meat and cheese favorites. Daily saturated fat limits: women, 12 g; men, 15 g.*

Instead of . . .	. . . Try Soy	Saturated Fat Savings Per Serving
Armour Homestyle Italian Meatballs	Veggitinos Wholesome Vegetable Meatballs	9 g
Weaver Chicken Nuggets	Morningstar Farms Chik Nuggets	3 g
Stouffer's Five Cheese Lasagna	Amy's Tofu Vegetable Lasagna	5 g
Red Baron Four Cheese Pizza	Amy's Organic Crust & Tomatoes Pizza	4 g
Weaver Hot Wings	2 Morningstar Farms Buffalo Wings	2 g

Based on 1,500 calories per day for women; 2,000 calories per day for men.

- To save money, boil dried legumes or use a pressure cooker and freeze the extra portions.
- If you prefer canned beans, rinse and drain before using to reduce sodium.
- Mix white beans with drained tuna, chopped red onion, cooked macaroni, and vinegar and olive oil.
- Add white beans, quick-frozen spinach, and rounds of cooked Italian turkey sausage to reduced-sodium chicken broth for a quick and hearty soup.

MEAT, POULTRY, AND FISH

Buy these:

- Boneless, skinless chicken breasts
- Canned salmon and tuna
- Extra-lean ground beef or ground turkey
- Fish and seafood (frozen or fresh)
- Lean boneless pork chops
- Soy or veggie burgers

Tasty tips:

- Cut raw or leftover chicken breast into chunks. Sauté in 1 to 2 teaspoons of taco or fajita seasoning or jarred curry paste. Add sliced raw onions and peppers and continue to sauté until the veggies are soft. Serve on salad greens and top with salsa and a dollop of fat-free sour cream (optional). You can use leftover pork chops or extra-lean ground beef or turkey, too.
- Here's another great way to use a leftover chicken breast or pork chop. All you need is a package of whole wheat wonton wrappers (available in natural food stores). Preheat the oven to 350°F. Shred chicken (there should be enough for 2 wrappers). Place lengthwise in wrappers, roll, and seal. Coat an ovenproof baking dish with olive or canola oil spray. Bake for 15 to 20 minutes, until the wrappers are crisp. Enjoy plain or with salsa, reduced-sodium soy sauce, or chutney. Makes 1 serving.
- To avoid exposure to mercury and PCB contaminents common to oily fish, choose light tuna packed in water (instead of albacore) and wild salmon (versus farmed).

- For salmon patties, mix drained, flaked salmon with chopped onion and a beaten egg white. Add enough fresh whole wheat bread crumbs to make a moist, but not runny, mixture. Form into patties and sauté in a nonstick skillet with a little olive oil until brown on both sides and heated through.
- Have a bit of leftover salmon? Cut it in chunks and toss with hot whole grain pasta, a tablespoon of olive oil, and fresh garlic. Even better if you have a handful of grape or cherry tomatoes toss them in, too.

NUTS

Buy these:

- 1 to 2 varieties of your favorite nuts; choose from the following: almonds, Brazil nuts, hazelnuts, peanuts, walnuts

Tasty tips:

- Try a wide variety of nuts—you'll diversify your health benefits. For example, walnuts contain heart-healthy omega-3s. And most varieties of nuts—including walnuts, almonds, peanuts, and hazelnuts—contain beta sitosterol and campesterol, two chemicals that can lower harmful blood cholesterol levels.
- To reduce your sodium intake, choose unsalted nuts.
- For the best flavor, toast almonds or walnuts lightly in a heavy skillet.
- Add 1 tablespoon of nuts to cooked vegetables, tossed salads, or grains.
- Nuts pack plenty of calories—about 180 calories an ounce—so keep portion sizes small (one handful equals 1 serving or 1 ounce).

CONDIMENTS, HERBS, AND SPICES

Buy these:

You already may have many of these items, but check your spice rack to see if you need to restock—or try something new.

- Basic seasonings: bay leaves, cinnamon, cumin (whole seeds), Italian seasoning, nutmeg, oregano, paprika, parsley (dried and fresh), rosemary, thyme
- Capers
- Chili sauce
- Cooking wine
- Dijon mustard
- Flax oil (store in the refrigerator)
- Horseradish
- Hot-pepper sauce
- Low-sodium soy sauce
- Natural sweeteners: honey, apple butter
- Olive and canola oils
- Salsa
- Sun-dried tomatoes
- Tahini
- Vinegars: balsamic, red wine, rice wine
- Worcestershire sauce

Sweet Success

JASON HENDERSON

Before he graduated from college with a major in wildlife management, Jason Henderson, 31, was at his perfect weight. At 5 feet 11 inches, he weighed between 180 and 185 pounds. After college, however, the Virginia resident realized his true calling and enrolled at the prestigious Culinary Institute of America in Hyde Park, New York. "I developed a taste for high-fat, high-sugar foods," says Jason. "And while the life of a chef can be tough, there isn't much exercise involved."

After graduating from culinary school in 1998, Jason found work as a chef in Germany. "The fats and carbs were plentiful, and the beer flowed freely," he says. By 2001, when he returned to the United States, he was 15 to 20 pounds heavier. Two and a half years later, when he started working for the army as an executive chef and analyst, he weighed in at 215 pounds.

On New Year's Day 2004, he stepped on the scale: He weighed 230 pounds. "It blew my mind," he says. He lost 20 pounds in 20 days on a low-carbohydrate diet. But then his weight loss stalled, and over the next year, he gained back 6 pounds.

In 2005, stuck at 216 pounds, Jason decided to try again. But this time, he traded in the no-carb approach for the slow-carb approach.

He ate six times a day to keep his blood sugar on an even keel, and he selected foods packed with fiber and slow carbs. Breakfast was oatmeal mixed with protein powder and applesauce. Lunch was a salad with lean meat, chicken, or fish. Dinner might be a peanut butter sandwich on whole grain bread, a portion of whole wheat pasta, or a serving of lean meat and vegetables. Between meals, Jason snacked on low-carbohydrate bars and smoothies made with fresh berries and low-fat milk or yogurt. He also started to exercise, lifting weights and pedaling an elliptical trainer two or three times a week.

Three months later, Jason was 26 pounds lighter. "Now I maintain at around 190 pounds, plus or minus a pound or two," he says. He still hits the gym and the cardio machines two to three times a week.

And he's maintained his weight in spite of being a chef. "Even working around food every day, I'm able to find foods that fit my way of eating," says Jason. "Some days, I find myself looking at my watch and saying, 'It's time to eat again?' My plan now is eating to live rather than living to eat."

CHAPTER 4

FREQUENTLY ASKED QUESTIONS

W hile individual results will vary among people who adopt any eating program, the same questions seem to come up for a lot of people. Ann Fittante, MS, RD, a certified diabetes educator, offers the answers that can help.

1. I'm 41 and have 40 pounds to lose. I follow the program exactly, but the weight is coming off very slowly. What's going on?

Lots of factors affect how quickly a woman in general—and you in particular—loses weight, including gender and age. Somewhere in her 30s, a woman's metabolism slows about 5 percent every decade. That means if a moderately active 35-year-old woman ate a set number of calories a day to maintain a weight of 140 pounds, she might gain weight eating the same number of calories at age 45. For many midlife women, the gain is so gradual they don't notice it until they step into their jeans and struggle with the zipper.

Though you're losing more slowly than you'd like, don't give up. Gradual weight loss is actually healthier, and most women who lose more slowly are more likely to keep that weight lost for good.

An average daily intake between 1,400 and 1,600 calories a day is an amount that helps most women lose weight. But to speed things up, consider increasing your daily physical activity by 100 to 200 calories a day. We're not talking much activity here. For example, if you're 155 pounds, you'll burn over 200 calories in 30 minutes of swimming.

If walking is your thing, you'll burn about 250 calories just walking the dog for an hour. (If you weigh more than 155 pounds, you'll burn more calories; less than 155 pounds, you'll burn fewer.)

You can also eliminate 200 to 300 calories each day. For example, you might eat smaller portions at dinner and eliminate one snack. But I recommend moving more. As I've said elsewhere, don't starve yourself. Consuming less than 1,200 calories a day will slow your metabolism even more.

2. I love my muffin in the morning. Any suggestions on how to make muffins acceptable on this program?

You bet! You're right to look for an alternative to store-bought muffins. Most are made with white flour and unhealthy trans fats. And if they're as big as softballs, which most of them are, they contain huge amounts of fat and calories.

For a muffin that won't wreak havoc on your insulin and blood sugar levels, try the Peanut Butter and Banana Streusel Muffins on page 46. Or if you'd rather, modify your favorite muffin recipe. Simply substitute half the flour with 100 percent whole wheat flour, reduce the sugar from 1 cup to ¾ cup, and use heart-healthy canola oil. You can also add nuts and/or ¼ cup of ground flaxseed.

3. On this program, I'm never hungry, and the menu plans are delicious. But the week before my period, I crave sweets, especially chocolate. Every month, I indulge and gain back a pound or two. What can I do to fight off these cravings and stick to the program?

It's fine to indulge in a small square of cake or a scoop of real, creamy ice cream now and then, especially when you're premenstrual. To master your monthly cravings for sweets without derailing your weight loss, calculate the caloric value of the treat you crave, and adjust your menu accordingly. For example, ½ cup of ice cream runs about 150 calories.

To accommodate those additional calories, eliminate one or two of your snacks during the day and/or have smaller portions at mealtime.

Here are a few other sweet treats that'll cost you 150 calories or less. Remember, these are "break glass in case of emergency" treats; they're not for everyday consumption.

- 2 Famous Amos Chocolate Chip Cookies (75 calories)
- 2 tablespoons of chocolate chips (140 calories)
- 4 chocolate kisses (105 calories)
- 2 ounces of angel food cake topped with fresh berries (73 calories)

Better yet, make your own healthier sweet treats. My personal favorite: the Oatmeal-Date Bars on page 168.

4. Is it true that consuming artificially sweetened drinks can lead to weight gain? Are they okay to drink on The Sugar Solution program?

Some studies have speculated that artificial sweeteners might stimulate hunger, while others suggested that sucrose (table sugar) might promote weight loss. To find out, Danish researchers asked 41 overweight people to supplement their diets with either sucrose or artificially sweetened drinks. Ten weeks later, the sucrose group gained an average of 3 pounds, while the fake-sweetener group lost nearly 2 pounds. Turns out the sucrose group added more than 400 calories each day to their normal intake. Calories you drink don't help satisfy your appetite. Because you never compensate for the extra calories by eating less, you end up gaining weight.

I think it's fine to consume artificially sweetened drinks in moderation. In my view, however, water is the way to go. Try one of the new, zero-calorie flavored waters, or mix an ounce of your favorite juice into a tall glass of ice water or club soda.

As far as artificially sweetened foods are concerned, check labels carefully. Many sugar-free foods, including cookies and ice cream, have calorie amounts similar to those of the regular brands and are high in unhealthy saturated and/or hydrogenated fats.

5. My husband and I would like to diet together—we both have about 30 pounds to lose. Does The Sugar Solution diet work for men, and does it meet their nutritional and caloric needs?

Yes, the recipes in this book meet nutritional requirements for both men and women. And how wonderful that you've partnered up! There's no doubt that you'll both lose weight (although he might lose a bit more quickly than you will—men usually do, because of their increased muscle mass).

While women usually lose weight when they stay between 1,400 and 1,600 calories, most men can lose weight on up to 1,800 calories a day. That's because men's bodies tend to be bigger and pack more calorie-burning muscle than women's. So if your husband feels very hungry, he can either eat larger portions at mealtime or enjoy a few healthy snacks.

6. I absolutely cannot live without bread, pasta, and potatoes. Is there any way I can enjoy them on the diet?

Yes! The Sugar Solution way of eating isn't about eating less but eating smart—and whole grain breads and pastas give your body the slow carbs it needs. Whole grains make your body work harder during digestion, which slows the rise in blood sugar. When blood sugar levels rise and fall gradually, you feel fuller longer and tend not to eat as often.

What's more, whole grain breads and pastas contain more fiber, iron, thiamin, and niacin than the processed kinds, cost only pennies more, and are now widely available in most large supermarkets. Opt for whole grain products that are 140 calories or less per serving and contain 3 or more grams of fiber per serving.

Potatoes are a good source of B-vitamins and potassium and also contain vitamin C and magnesium. Just eat them in sensible portions (one small baked potato, for example) with low-fat toppings like salsa, cottage cheese, or low-fat sour cream. Eat the skin, too—it's a good source of fiber. Better yet, upgrade your carbs and enjoy a sweet potato instead of a white potato.

7. What can I use instead of butter for cooking, on bread, and on vegetables?

I'm glad you recognize that although butter is a zero-carbohydrate food, it's still a saturated fat, which can raise cholesterol levels. I recommend it as a treat rather than as an everyday part of your diet. To reduce its saturated fat content, blend it with canola oil. Use one part canola oil to one part butter (for example, ¼ cup of canola oil blended with ¼ cup of butter). Also, feel free to use one of those butter-flavor sprays that mimic the taste of butter without the fat or calories.

I'm a big fan of olive or canola oil on—and in—just about any food, in place of butter or margarine. Olive oil, in particular, adds flavor without the heart-damaging saturated fats. I love to sauté my veggies in olive oil and garlic and dip my whole grain bread in olive oil. When I bake, I use canola oil.

8. I have a family history of obesity and diabetes, and my 15-year-old daughter is about 25 pounds overweight. Is it safe for her to go on the program? I want to help her protect her future health.

The Sugar Solution isn't designed to meet the nutritional needs of teenagers (or children or pregnant women, either). Their calorie needs are quite high: between 1,800 and 3,000 calories per day for teenage girls, and even more for teenage boys. It's generally healthier for teens not to restrict calories but to reduce the number of empty calories they consume in the form of soda, sweets, chips, and fast foods. Although I can't recommend that your teen follow the program itself, the recipes, of course, are healthful choices for the entire family.

9. Can I still eat fruit? I enjoy it, but I've read that it can slow weight loss because it increases insulin and blood sugar levels.

I don't know where these rumors get started. Fruit does not slow weight loss. Consuming too many calories and/or not exercising regularly does. Nor does fruit increase insulin or blood sugar levels to unhealthy levels. An average-size piece of fruit contains between 15 and 30 grams of carbohydrate. To manage blood sugars, I generally recommend that people with diabetes or insulin resistance consume between 30 and 60 grams of carbohydrate for meals and between 15 and 30 grams of carbohydrate for snacks.

Bottom line: Enjoy from 1 to 3 servings of fruit a day. A medium-size piece contains 100 calories or less and loads of fiber and important vitamins.

10. Like many women, I overeat when I'm stressed. The problem is, I'm stressed out every day! I try to be good, but food calms me. How can I put the brakes on my stress eating?

In prehistoric times, anxious eating may have been a smart survival strategy. Your agitated ancestors grabbed berries after the marauding tigers slunk away; you head for the candy machine after the boss roars. Research has found that stress prompts rats to release hormone signals for high-calorie eating, and it may be similar in humans.

Have you begun The Sugar Solution program? If not, you're bound to discover what many women and men who follow it have already learned: Eating sensible portions of high-fiber, nutritionally balanced food every few hours—rather than skipping meals and gorging on fatty, sugary junk—helps control physiological hunger. You may just find that although your stress level stays the same, your urge to eat your way through stressful situations is drastically reduced. More good news: Exercise, sleep, and healthy eating may keep the stress/eat cycle from kicking in. Try a brisk, 10-minute walk or other stress-busting technique to help break the stress-gorging habit.

11. Do I have to exercise on The Sugar Solution program?

Everyone needs regular exercise, and improved fitness can do more for your body than speed up weight loss. It can also reduce insulin resistance and boost energy.

Cardiovascular exercise—cardio, for short—elevates your metabolism before and after exercise. Resistance training increases muscle mass, which in turn increases the body's ability to burn calories both during activity and at rest.

But before you lace up your walking shoes or heft a dumbbell, get your doctor's okay to exercise. Then choose an activity that you enjoy. Start at 30 minutes and work up to 60 minutes of activity, three to six times a week. Begin slowly and increase as your body becomes more fit.

12. I want to try *The Sugar Solution*, but I don't think I can eat six times a day. I'm not hungry at breakfast, usually work through lunch, and eat one meal a day: dinner. Do I really have to eat all these meals?

At least give it a try, because skipping meals has derailed many a dieter's weight-loss efforts. Not eating at regular intervals leads to low blood sugar, which leads to hunger and cravings, which leads to binging. On the other hand, spacing meals and snacks evenly throughout the day helps maintain better blood sugar control and prevent overeating. And we're not talking about large meals here—half a turkey sandwich and a piece of fruit, a small grilled-chicken salad, a low-fat yogurt, and a couple of whole grain crackers. These mini-meals are easy to stash in your desk or the refrigerator at work, and they're easy to find in convenience stores, too.

If you just can't manage six times a day, try eating at least three times a day for two weeks. Chances are, you'll have more energy during the day and feel less hungry by evening.

13. Do you suggest taking supplements while on the program?

On The Sugar Solution program, you'll eat nutrient-dense fruits, veggies, and whole grains and modest amounts of low-fat dairy products and lean meat, poultry, and fish. Still, taking a multivitamin is nutritional insurance—one that *Prevention* recommends for everyone. In fact, a panel of nutrition experts recently concluded that all adults should take a multi. Assuming that you take a multi and eat a healthy diet like The Sugar Solution, you're pretty well covered.

Along with a multi (which should contain 400 IU of vitamin D), consider taking 500 mg of calcium as a separate supplement up to age 50. Over 50, consider taking 700 mg separately but not more than 500 mg at a time for best absorption.

Although I believe that supplements can help meet nutritional requirements, I suggest that you avoid the multivitamin supplements marketed to people on low-carbohydrate diets or any other supplement that claims to promote weight loss. They don't work, and they're a waste of your hard-earned money.

14. I dislike the taste and texture of whole wheat pasta. Can I mix regular pasta with the whole grain kind? Or can you suggest another type of whole grain noodle with a taste and texture more like regular pasta?

Many people who swore they'd never give up white flour pasta have come to love the distinctive taste of the whole wheat variety. (It's chewier than pasta made with white flour, with a nutlike flavor.) But if you can't quite manage whole wheat pasta by itself, it's fine to mix it with white pasta.

Your local health food store will contain a variety of whole grain pastas, including those made with corn, quinoa, spelt, and brown rice. You may enjoy the taste and texture of these varieties better.

15. Can I use condiments on the program, like ketchup, barbecue sauce, and relish?

Yes, you can use condiments—just don't go overboard. One tablespoon is considered free and will not contribute greatly to calories, fat, or sodium. But I encourage you to experiment with alternatives to conventional condiments, or use lower-calorie condiments. For example, salsa is delicious on burgers or scrambled eggs, and I know of people who top their baked potatoes with spicy brown mustard!

16. I'm a night eater. I follow the program until 8 p.m. By 11, I've eaten hundreds of extra calories, and my waistline shows it. What can I do?

It's important to identify the reasons for late-night eating. Are you hungry? Are you bored? Or is noshing at night simply a habit? Make sure that your night eating isn't a physiological response to hunger. The large majority of people who struggle with night eating are those who skip meals or don't eat balanced meals during the day. This is a major setup for overeating at night. If you stick to The Sugar Solution formula of three meals and three snacks a day, chances are that you want to eat for reasons other than physiological hunger.

I'd advise you to practice mindful eating—that is, pay attention to what, how, and how much you eat, as well as your sense of fullness or hunger. To eat mindfully, you need to do nothing when you eat but eat—that means don't watch TV, read, or work. The following exercise, which takes all of about 3 minutes, can help you understand what mindful eating is all about.

Place a finger food in your palm—a nugget of cereal, a grape, a baby carrot. Then pick it up with your fingers. Focus on its shape and texture. Think about this piece of food—where it came from, how it grew. Put it into your mouth, but don't bite it: Simply let it stay in your mouth. Roll it around. Explore it with your tongue. Finally, chew it slowly, focusing on its flavor.

It also might help you to plan an activity for after 8 p.m. You might practice meditation or relaxation techniques or a hobby like needlepoint, knitting, or drawing. If all else fails, simply draw a bath, or step into the shower. It's tough to eat with wet hands or nails.

17. I love a glass of wine with dinner. Can I drink alcohol on this program?

Yes. Just be aware that alcohol tends to raise cortisol levels, sending fat to your belly, and the extra calories could slow your weight loss if you don't plan for them. One drink (which equals 4 ounces of wine, 12 ounces of beer, or 1 ounce of hard liquor) contains from 80 to 150 calories. Eliminate one or two snacks during the day, or have smaller portions at mealtime. For health reasons, women should have no more than one alcoholic beverage per day (men, no more than two a day).

Another reason to cut back on drinking: One study found that, compared with juice or water, having one alcoholic drink before a meal led to eating 200 extra calories—on top of the added calories in the drink itself. Subjects ate faster, took longer to feel full, and continued eating even after they were no longer hungry.

18. I don't have time to cook all these meals. What should I do?

It's true that preparing meals involves more time and energy than picking up a pizza or hitting the drive-through. But not much more time, especially if you plan. Dedicate 1 to 2

Sweet Success

HELEN LEVELS

From the time she was a girl, Helen Levels craved cookies, cake, and candy. But these treats were off-limits. "My parents wouldn't let us kids have anything sweet, except fruit," recalls the 52-year-old San Antonio resident.

Then her mother passed away, and 13-year-old Helen moved in with an aunt whose dietary guidelines were less restrictive. Finally, Helen could indulge her sweet tooth—and indulge she did! Thus began a 22-year love affair with sweets.

After she married her husband, Bruce, and started a family, Helen's sweet tooth remained as active as ever. Unfortunately, her body didn't, and the pounds began to pile on. Having honey buns slathered with butter and sugar for breakfast and bowls of ice cream or frozen yogurt for lunch didn't help. At her heaviest, she carried 193 pounds on her 5-foot-2 frame.

When Helen turned 35, her normally boundless energy drained away. "I didn't have the energy to do anything," she says. "After work, I'd go home, collapse on the couch, and sleep." She was always thirsty, drinking three 32-ounce bottles of water a day and running to the bathroom two or three times in a half hour. More ominously, Helen lost 30 pounds.

One day, she took a bite of cheesecake a neighbor had made and became so tired, "I didn't think I'd make it to the couch." The next day, Bruce took her to the emergency room. She told the doctors her symptoms: fatigue, thirst, frequent urination. They tested her blood sugar. The results: diabetes.

"The doctors said, 'You have to start eating better and exercising now,'" Helen recalls. Alarmed, she immediately replaced the quick-carb sweets in her diet with nutritious, slow-carb fare. Breakfast became a small bowl of bran flakes with milk. Lunch was soup, salad, or fruit salad. On her dinner menu: chicken or fish.

At first, her sweet tooth rebelled. "Sometimes I wanted something sweet so badly I thought I would cry," she says. But her determination—and fear—kept her cookie free.

Helen also purchased a treadmill. Each night after work, she walked—just 15 minutes at first, increasing to an hour over the course of several months.

Within a year, Helen's energy was back and her blood sugar readings vastly improved—without medication. "This morning, my blood sugar was 98 mg/dl," she says. Best of all, Helen lost 43 pounds, now weighing in at 150 pounds. "And I don't crave sweets anymore," she says.

What Helen does crave is staying healthy. "Too many people around me—people younger than I am—are getting sick or dying of diabetes," she says. "I don't want to go through that. If it takes giving up sweets to stay in good health, I'm willing to give them up."

hours a week to meal planning. Set aside an evening or weekend day to preparing more time-intensive meals such as casseroles, muffins or quick breads, soups, and stews. Try to incorporate one new recipe per week. Cook double batches of favorite recipes so you can freeze the unused portion or have leftovers.

Keep in mind that The Sugar Solution is a *lifelong* program that helps you keep off those extra pounds for good. Would you rather save time picking up a bucket of chicken, or look smashing in a smaller pair of jeans?

HEARTY, SUGAR-BALANCING BREAKFASTS

FAST   SUPER FAST   FAST PREP

ZUCCHINI AND DILL FRITTATA

Photo on page 89.

Prep time: 10 minutes • Cook time: 14 minutes

2 teaspoons butter

2 cups finely chopped zucchini (one 8-ounce zucchini)

2 large scallions, thinly sliced

4 eggs

6 egg whites

1 tablespoon water

2 tablespoons chopped fresh dill

¼ teaspoon freshly ground black pepper

3 tablespoons grated Parmesan cheese

Preheat the broiler. Heat a 10" nonstick skillet over medium heat. Add the butter and zucchini. Cook for 5 minutes, stirring occasionally. Stir in the scallions and cook for 3 minutes more, or until the zucchini is just tender.

Meanwhile, in a medium bowl, whisk together the eggs, egg whites, water, dill, pepper, and 2 tablespoons of the cheese. Add to the skillet and cook for 5 minutes, occasionally lifting the edges of the egg mixture with a spatula and tilting the pan, allowing the uncooked mixture to flow underneath. (The eggs will be set on the bottom but will still be moist on the top.) Remove from the heat and sprinkle on the remaining 1 tablespoon cheese.

Wrap the skillet handle with a double thickness of foil. Broil 4" from the heat for 1 to 2 minutes, or until the eggs are set on the top. Cut into quarters and serve immediately.

Makes 4 servings

Per serving: 148 calories, 14 g protein, 4 g carbohydrates, 8 g fat, 220 mg cholesterol, 220 mg sodium, 1 g dietary fiber
Diet Exchanges: 2 meat, 1 fat
Carb Choices: 0

CARROT CAKE PANCAKES WITH MAPLE–CREAM CHEESE SPREAD

Prep time: 25 minutes • Cook time: 15 minutes

SPREAD

3 ounces Neufchâtel cheese, at room temperature

2 tablespoons maple syrup + additional for serving

$^1/_4$ teaspoon ground cinnamon

PANCAKES

$^1/_4$ cup walnuts, halved

1 cup shredded carrot

$1^1/_2$ cups whole grain pastry flour

$^3/_4$ cup unbleached or all-purpose flour

2 teaspoons baking powder

$1^1/_4$ teaspoons ground cinnamon

$^1/_4$ teaspoon ground allspice

$^1/_4$ teaspoon salt

$1^1/_2$ cups soymilk

$^1/_3$ cup packed brown sugar

3 egg whites

2 tablespoons canola oil

To make the spread: In a medium bowl, stir together the Neufchâtel, maple syrup, and cinnamon until blended. Set aside.

To make the pancakes: Preheat the oven to 300°F. Spread the walnuts on a baking sheet and toast just until fragrant, 5 minutes or longer. Chop the nuts and set aside.

Meanwhile, place the carrot in a small microwaveable bowl. Cover loosely with plastic wrap and microwave on high power for 1 minute, or until just tender. Set aside to cool.

In a large bowl, whisk together the whole grain flour, all-purpose flour, baking powder, cinnamon, allspice, salt, and walnuts until blended. Make a well in the center of the flour mixture. Add the milk, sugar, egg whites, and oil and whisk the ingredients together until blended. Add the cooled carrot and stir just until blended.

Preheat a large nonstick skillet or griddle over medium-high heat and coat with cooking spray. Ladle $^1/_4$ cup batter for each pancake and cook for 2 minutes, or until bubbles form on the surface.

Flip with a spatula and cook for 1 minute longer, or until cooked through. (Keep warm in the preheated oven, if needed.) To serve, spoon a rounded teaspoon of the maple cream cheese spread on each pancake and drizzle with additional maple syrup, if you wish.

Makes 12 to 14 pancakes, $^1/_2$ cup maple-cream cheese spread

Per pancake: 171 calories, 5 g protein, 25 g carbohydrates, 7 g fat, 5 mg cholesterol, 180 mg sodium, 2 g dietary fiber
Diet Exchanges: 2 bread, 1 meat, 1 fat
Carb Choices: 2

PANCAKE AND WAFFLE TOPPINGS

Pancakes are an American classic. Try this simple fruit topping to jazz up your plain pancakes and waffles and enjoy a naturally sweet start to your morning.

APPLE TOPPING

    3 cups thinly sliced peeled apples

    2 tablespoons apple or white grape juice

    2 tablespoons honey

 $^1/_8$ teaspoon ground nutmeg

In a medium saucepan over low heat, add the apples, juice, honey, and nutmeg. Cook, stirring occasionally, for 3 minutes. Cover the pan and cook for 5 minutes, or until the fruit is softened. Cool slightly before serving.

Note: This topping can be reheated on top of the stove or in the microwave. Try peaches instead of apples, too.

Makes 2 cups. Per $^1/_2$ cup: 85 calories, 0.2 g protein, 22 g carbohydrates, 0.3 g fat, 0 mg cholesterol, 1 mg sodium, 1.9 g dietary fiber

BERRY SAUCE

 $2 ^1/_4$ cups fresh or frozen mixed berries

    2 tablespoons water

    2 tablespoons honey

 $^1/_4$ teaspoon freshly grated citrus rind
       (optional)

In a small saucepan over low heat, combine the berries, water, honey, and rind, if using. Cook, stirring occasionally, for 8 minutes, or until the berry juices are released.

Puree in a food processor or blender. Pass through a sieve to remove the seeds.

Return the mixture to the saucepan. Cook over medium heat for 3 minutes, or until the sauce is reduced to about 1 cup. Cool.

Makes 1 cup. Per $^1/_4$ cup: 78 calories, 0.5 g protein, 20 g carbohydrates, 0.3 g fat, 0 mg cholesterol, 5 mg sodium, 2.2 g dietary fiber

PEANUT BUTTER AND BANANA STREUSEL MUFFINS

Photo on page 90.

Prep time: 15 minutes • Cook time: 16 minutes

STREUSEL

3 tablespoons whole grain pastry flour

3 tablespoons packed brown sugar

1 tablespoon butter, melted

1 teaspoon honey

MUFFINS

2 cups whole grain pastry flour

2 teaspoons baking powder

1 teaspoon ground cinnamon

½ teaspoon salt

½ cup pureed ripe banana (about 1 medium banana)

½ cup unsweetened applesauce

⅓ cup peanut butter

½ cup packed brown sugar

1 egg

¾ cup 1% milk

1 teaspoon vanilla extract

Preheat the oven to 400°F. Coat a 12-cup muffin pan with cooking spray.

To make the streusel: In a small bowl, stir together the flour, sugar, butter, and honey with a spoon until the mixture forms wet crumbs.

To make the muffins: In a medium bowl, whisk together the flour, baking powder, cinnamon, and salt until combined. In a large bowl, whisk together the banana, applesauce, peanut butter, sugar, and egg until blended. Whisk the milk and vanilla into the banana mixture until combined.

Stir the flour mixture into the banana mixture with a spoon, just until blended. Do not overmix. Spoon the batter into the prepared muffin cups, dividing evenly. Crumble the streusel mixture on top of the muffin batter, dividing evenly.

Bake for 16 to 18 minutes, or until a wooden pick inserted in the center of a muffin comes out clean. Remove from the pan and serve warm.

Makes 18

Per muffin: 93 calories, 3 g protein, 13 g carbohydrates, 4 g fat, 15 mg cholesterol, 150 mg sodium, 2 g dietary fiber
Diet Exchanges: 1 bread, 1 fat
Carb Choices: 1

WHOLE GRAIN IRISH SODA BREAD

Prep time: 15 minutes • Cook time: 40 minutes

⅓ cup golden raisins	1 teaspoon baking soda
⅓ cup dried currants	2 teaspoons caraway seeds (optional)
2 tablespoons apple juice or sherry	½ teaspoon salt
2 tablespoons butter	1⅓ cups buttermilk
2½ cups whole grain flour	1 egg
¾ cup + 1½ tablespoons oat flour	1 egg white
2 teaspoons baking powder	¼ cup packed brown sugar

Preheat the oven to 375°F. Coat a 9" springform pan or a 9" × 1" cake pan with cooking spray. Combine the raisins, currants, apple juice or sherry, and butter in a microwaveable dish. Cover loosely with plastic wrap and microwave on high power for 1 minute. Stir and set aside to cool.

In a large bowl, toss together the whole grain flour, the ¾ cup oat flour, baking powder, baking soda, caraway seeds (if using), and salt. In a medium bowl, whisk together the buttermilk, egg, egg white, and sugar until blended. Stir the raisin mixture into the egg mixture and then stir into the flour mixture just until combined. Do not overmix.

Pour into the prepared pan and spread to mound slightly in the center. Sprinkle the remaining 1½ tablespoons oat flour over the top. Slash a large X on the top of the bread using a sharp, flour-dipped knife.

Bake for 40 minutes, or until golden brown and a wooden pick inserted in the center comes out clean. Transfer to a rack to cool for at least 15 minutes. Cut into 16 wedges and serve warm or at room temperature.

Makes 16 servings

Per serving: 114 calories, 4 g protein, 20 g carbohydrates, 2 g fat, 20 mg cholesterol, 240 mg sodium, 2 g dietary fiber
Diet Exchanges: ½ fruit, 1 bread
Carb Choices: 1½

MINTED HONEY-LIME FRUIT SALAD

Photo on page 91.

Prep time: 20 minutes

1 teaspoon grated lime peel	$\frac{1}{2}$ small honeydew, cubed
2 tablespoons lime juice	$\frac{1}{2}$ cantaloupe, cubed
3–4 tablespoons honey (see note)	1 pint fresh strawberries, halved and hulled
3 tablespoons chopped fresh mint	2 cups fresh pineapple or mango cubes

In a large bowl, stir together the lime peel, juice, honey, and mint until combined. Add the honeydew, cantaloupe, strawberries, and pineapple or mango. Toss to combine.

Note: Depending on the sweetness of the fruit, start with 3 tablespoons honey, adding more honey if needed.

Makes 8 servings

Per serving: 92 calories, 1 g protein, 24 g carbohydrates, 0 g fat, 0 mg cholesterol, 30 mg sodium, 2 g dietary fiber
Diet Exchanges: 2 fruit
Carb Choices: 2

HEALTHY NIBBLES: SNACKS AND BEVERAGES

FAST   SUPER FAST   FAST PREP

ROASTED RED PEPPER HUMMUS WITH CILANTRO

Prep time: 20 minutes • **Cook time: 15 minutes** • **Stand time: 10 minutes**

2 red bell peppers

4 large cloves garlic, unpeeled

1 can (15 ½ ounces) chickpeas, rinsed and drained

2 tablespoons tahini

2 tablespoons lemon juice

1 tablespoon mild cayenne pepper sauce

¼ cup chopped fresh cilantro

   Assorted vegetable sticks, for dipping

Preheat the broiler. Place the peppers on a foil-lined baking sheet. Wrap the garlic in foil and place on the sheet. Broil the peppers 6" from the heat for 15 to 20 minutes, turning until charred on all sides. Broil the garlic for 15 minutes. Place the peppers in a sealed bag and let stand for 10 minutes.

Meanwhile, when it's cool enough to handle, peel the garlic and finely chop in a food processor. When the peppers are cool enough to handle, peel, core, and seed them. (You should have 1 cup of roasted peppers.) Add the peppers, chickpeas, tahini, lemon juice, and pepper sauce to the processor and blend until smooth. Add the cilantro and process just until combined. For best flavor, store refrigerated for at least 4 hours or up to 3 days. Serve with vegetable sticks or use as a spread for wraps or sandwiches.

Makes 4 servings (2 cups)

Per serving: 174 calories, 7 g protein, 27 g carbohydrates, 5 g fat, 0 mg cholesterol, 260 mg sodium, 6 g dietary fiber
Diet Exchanges: 1 vegetable, 1 ½ bread, 1 fat
Carb Choices: 2

ORANGE-DIJON MUSTARD DIP

Prep time: 10 minutes

¼ cup Dijon mustard

2 tablespoons frozen orange juice concentrate, thawed

¼ cup plain yogurt

2 tablespoons reduced-fat sour cream

½ teaspoon white wine vinegar

Mini whole wheat pretzels, for dipping

Assorted vegetable sticks, for dipping

In a medium bowl, stir together the mustard, orange juice concentrate, yogurt, sour cream, and vinegar until smooth. (Can be made ahead and refrigerated up to 4 days in advance.) Serve as a dip, along with pretzels and vegetable sticks.

Makes 4 servings (1 cup)

Per serving: 45 calories, 2 g protein, 4 g carbohydrates, 3 g fat, 5 mg cholesterol, 390 mg sodium, 0 g dietary fiber
Diet Exchanges: ½ fat
Carb Choices: 0

BUFFALO CHICKEN BITES

Photo on page 92.

Prep time: 25 minutes • Cook time: 15 minutes

BLUE CHEESE DRESSING

3 tablespoons (1 ¼ ounces) crumbled blue cheese

⅓ cup reduced-fat sour cream

2 teaspoons finely chopped green onion

½ teaspoon white wine vinegar

CHICKEN BITES

2 boneless, skinless chicken breast halves (10 ounces), cut into 1" cubes

1 scallion, finely chopped

2 ½ tablespoons mild cayenne pepper sauce

1 tablespoon butter, melted

3 ribs celery, cut into 2" sticks

1 cup baby carrots

To make the blue cheese dressing: In a small bowl, mash together the blue cheese and sour cream with the back of a spoon. Stir in the green onion and vinegar until blended. Set aside.

To make the chicken bites: Preheat the oven to 400°F. In a medium bowl, toss together the chicken cubes, scallion, and 1 tablespoon of the pepper sauce. Thread the chicken on twelve 6" bamboo skewers, using 2 pieces of chicken per skewer. Arrange on a foil-lined baking sheet. Bake for 15 minutes, or until cooked through.

Meanwhile, in a small bowl, toss together the remaining 1 ½ tablespoons pepper sauce and the butter. Arrange the cooked chicken skewers on one half of a serving platter in a single layer. Brush the chicken cubes with the pepper sauce. Place the celery and carrots on the platter and serve with the blue cheese dressing.

Makes 4 servings

Per serving: 200 calories, 20 g protein, 9 g carbohydrates, 9 g fat, 65 mg cholesterol, 260 mg sodium, 3 g dietary fiber
Diet Exchanges: 1 vegetable, 2 ½ meat, 1 ½ fat
Carb Choices: 1

CHOCOLATE MALTED MILKSHAKE

Photo on page 93.

SUPER FAST

Prep time: 10 minutes

¾ **cup vanilla frozen yogurt**

3 **tablespoons malted milk powder**

1½ **tablespoons cocoa powder**

½ **teaspoon instant espresso coffee powder**

1 **cup soymilk or 1% milk**

1 **teaspoon vanilla extract**

In a blender, combine the frozen yogurt, malted milk powder, cocoa, coffee powder, milk, and vanilla. Process until smooth. Pour into tall glasses and serve immediately.

Makes 2 servings (1 cup each)

Per serving: 257 calories, 8 g protein, 45 g carbohydrates, 7 g fat, 5 mg cholesterol, 140 mg sodium, 3 g dietary fiber
Diet Exchanges: 3 bread, ½ meat, 1 fat
Carb Choices: 3

STRAWBERRY-MANGO SMOOTHIE

Photo on page 93.

Prep time: 10 minutes

1½ **cups cubed fresh (about 1) or frozen mango**

2 **cups fresh strawberries + 2 berries for garnish**

1 **tablespoon minced candied ginger**

2 **tablespoons honey**

1 **cup cold soymilk or 1% milk**

Pinch of ground allspice

In a blender, combine the mango, strawberries, ginger, honey, soymilk or milk, and allspice. Process until smooth. Pour the mixture into 2 glasses and garnish with fresh strawberries.

Makes 2 servings (1½ cups each)

Per serving: 191 calories, 4 g protein, 42 g carbohydrates, 3 g fat, 20 mg cholesterol, 42 mg sodium, 4 g dietary fiber
Diet Exchanges: 1½ fruit, 1 bread, ½ meat, ½ fat
Carb Choices: 3

GAZPACHO-VEGGIE TWISTER

Prep time: 10 minutes

1¾ cups tomato juice or vegetable-tomato
cocktail

2 small (about 4") pickling cucumbers
(6 ounces), peeled and cubed

½ red bell pepper, peeled and cubed

½ rib celery, sliced

1 tablespoon lemon juice

2 teaspoons Worcestershire sauce

1 teaspoon green Tabasco sauce, or 6 drops
of regular Tabasco

Cucumber spears and lemon wedges
(optional)

In a blender, combine the tomato juice or vegetable-tomato cocktail, cucumbers, bell pepper,
celery, lemon juice, Worcestershire sauce, and Tabasco sauce. Process for 1 to 2 minutes, or until
smooth. Serve over ice. Garnish with cucumber spears and lemon wedges, if you wish.

Makes 2 servings (1½ cups each)

Per serving: 69 calories, 3 g protein, 14 g carbohydrates, 0 g fat, 0 mg cholesterol, 830 mg sodium, 2 g dietary fiber
Diet Exchanges: 2 ½ vegetable
Carb Choices: 1

CHAPTER 7

HEARTY SOUPS AND SANDWICHES

■ FAST ■ SUPER FAST ■ FAST PREP

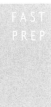

LENTIL SOUP WITH SPINACH

Prep time: 10 minutes • Cook time: 36 minutes

1 tablespoon olive oil	1 ⅓ cups (8 ounces) lentils, sorted and rinsed
1 ½ teaspoons whole cumin seeds	5 cups water
1 large onion, chopped	1 can (14 ½ ounces) diced tomatoes
4 cloves garlic, minced	2 cups packed shredded fresh spinach
½ teaspoon ground coriander	½ teaspoon salt
½ teaspoon freshly ground black pepper	8 ounces fat-free plain yogurt
1 teaspoon paprika	

Place the oil and cumin seeds in a Dutch oven or heavy large saucepan over medium heat. Cook, stirring, for 2 to 3 minutes, or until fragrant. Stir in the onion, garlic, coriander, and pepper and cook, stirring often, for 4 to 6 minutes, or until the onions and garlic are tender. Stir in the paprika.

Add the lentils and water. Cover and bring to a boil. Reduce the heat to low and simmer, covered, for 30 to 35 minutes, or until the lentils are very tender.

Stir in the diced tomatoes, spinach, and salt. Increase the heat and simmer, uncovered, for 5 minutes longer. Serve with a swirl of yogurt.

Makes 4 main-dish servings (7 ½ cups)

Per serving: 303 calories, 21 g protein, 50 g carbohydrates, 4 g fat, 0 mg cholesterol, 490 mg sodium, 21 g dietary fiber
Diet Exchanges: 2 vegetable, 2 bread, 2 meat, ½ fat
Carb Choices: 3

POTATO AND VEGETABLE SOUP

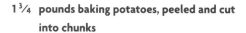

Prep time: 25 minutes • Cook time: 35 minutes

1¾ pounds baking potatoes, peeled and cut into chunks

1 large onion, sliced

2 ribs celery with leaves, sliced

5 cups chicken broth

2 cups water

½ teaspoon dried thyme, crumbled

2 tablespoons olive oil

3 cups sliced cremini or baby portobello mushrooms

1 large leek, halved lengthwise, well washed, and cut into ½" slices

2 large carrots, cut into ¼" slices

2 cups small broccoli florets

1 medium yellow summer squash, sliced lengthwise and cut into ¼" slices

½ teaspoon salt

¼ teaspoon freshly ground black pepper

1 cup 1% milk

Place the potatoes, onion, celery, broth, water, and thyme in a Dutch oven. Cover and bring to a boil over high heat.

Reduce the heat to low and simmer, covered, for 20 to 25 minutes, or until the potatoes and celery are very tender. In a food processor, puree the potatoes and celery to a smooth consistency.

Meanwhile, in a heavy large, deep skillet, heat the oil over medium heat. Add the mushrooms, leek, carrots, broccoli, and squash. Sprinkle with salt and pepper, mix well, and reduce the heat to low. Cover and cook, stirring occasionally, for 10 minutes, or until the vegetables are nearly tender.

Add the vegetables and milk to the potato mixture. Stir to blend, and bring to a simmer over medium-high heat. Cook, stirring often, for 5 minutes, or until the vegetables are very tender.

Makes 6 main-dish servings (14 cups)

Per serving: 239 calories, 10 g protein, 41 g carbohydrates, 7 g fat, 0 mg cholesterol, 1,090 mg sodium, 7 g dietary fiber
Diet Exchanges: 3 vegetable, 1½ bread, ½ meat, 1 fat
Carb Choices: 3

SPICY CORN AND SWEET POTATO CHOWDER

Prep time: 20 minutes • Cook time: 27 minutes

1   **tablespoon olive oil**

1   **large onion, coarsely chopped**

1   **red bell pepper, coarsely chopped**

2   **ribs celery, chopped**

¼   **teaspoon salt**

¼   **teaspoon freshly ground black pepper**

1½   **teaspoons ground cumin**

¼   **teaspoon dried oregano**

1   **large sweet potato (1 pound), peeled and cut into ½" chunks**

1   **package (10 ounces) frozen corn**

4   **cups chicken broth**

½   **cup medium-spicy salsa + extra for serving**

½   **ripe avocado, peeled and chopped**

½   **cup coarsely chopped fresh cilantro (optional)**

In a Dutch oven, warm the oil over medium-low heat. Add the onion, bell pepper, celery, salt, and black pepper. Cover and cook, stirring often, for 10 minutes, or until tender. Stir in the cumin and oregano.

Add the sweet potato, corn, and broth. Cover, increase the heat, and bring to a boil. Lower the heat and simmer, covered, for 12 minutes, or until the sweet potato is tender. Stir in the salsa and simmer, uncovered, for 5 minutes longer.

Ladle into bowls and top each with some of the avocado, cilantro (if using), and extra salsa, if you wish.

Makes 8 first-course servings (9 cups)

Per serving: 161 calories, 4 g protein, 30 g carbohydrates, 5 g fat, 0 mg cholesterol, 680 mg sodium, 5 g dietary fiber
Diet Exchanges: 1 vegetable, 1½ bread, 1 fat
Carb Choices: 2

PEPPER STEAK SOUP

Photo on page 94.

Prep time: 20 minutes • Cook time: 25 minutes

FAST
PREP

12 ounces well-trimmed lean boneless beef top round

½ teaspoon salt

½ teaspoon coarsely ground black pepper

4 cups fat-free beef broth

½ cup dry red wine (optional)

½ cup tomato sauce

¼ teaspoon dried thyme

1 tablespoon olive oil

1 medium sweet white onion, halved and thinly sliced

2 green bell peppers, cut into strips

4 cloves garlic, minced

3 tablespoons water

1½ cups halved cherry tomatoes

Thinly slice the beef on the diagonal into ¼"-thick slices. Cut large pieces in half. Sprinkle with ¼ teaspoon of the salt and the black pepper. Set aside.

In a large saucepan, stir together the beef broth, wine (if using), tomato sauce, and thyme. Cover and bring to a boil over high heat. Reduce the heat to low and simmer, covered, for 10 minutes.

Meanwhile, in a large nonstick skillet, warm the oil over medium-high heat until hot but not smoking. Add half the beef slices and cook, turning once, for 2 minutes, or until browned. Transfer to a clean bowl. Cook the remaining beef.

Add the onion, bell peppers, garlic, and the remaining ¼ teaspoon salt to the skillet. Toss to mix well and add 2 tablespoons of the water. Lower the heat to medium and cook, stirring often, for 10 minutes, or until the vegetables are tender. If the pan gets dry, add the remaining 1 tablespoon water. Add the tomatoes and cook, stirring often, for 5 minutes, or until softened.

Add the beef and any juices and the vegetables to the broth mixture. Warm through but don't boil.

Makes 4 main-dish servings (8 to 10 cups)

Per serving: 230 calories, 26 g protein, 15 g carbohydrates, 7 g fat, 50 mg cholesterol, 670 mg sodium, 3 g dietary fiber
Diet Exchanges: 2 vegetable, 3½ meat, 1 fat
Carb Choices: 1

BEEF BARLEY SOUP WITH MUSHROOMS

Prep time: 25 minutes • Cook time: 1 hour 40 minutes

1 tablespoon olive oil

1 pound well-trimmed lean boneless beef top round, cut into ³/₄" cubes

2 medium onions, halved and thinly sliced

3 cloves garlic, minced

³/₄ teaspoon salt

¹/₄ teaspoon freshly ground black pepper

¹/₂ teaspoon dried thyme, crumbled

10 ounces cremini or baby portobello mushrooms, sliced

2 ribs celery with some leaves, thinly sliced

2 medium carrots, sliced

1 medium parsnip, halved lengthwise and sliced

3 cups water

3 ¹/₂ cups fat-free beef broth

¹/₂ cup pearl barley

Chopped fresh parsley or dill (optional)

Heat the oil in a Dutch oven or a heavy large saucepan over medium heat. Add the beef cubes. Lightly brown the beef until the liquid evaporates. Add the onions and garlic and cook for 3 to 5 minutes, or until the onions soften. Add the salt, pepper, and thyme and cook for 1 minute. Add the mushrooms and cook for 3 minutes, or until the mushrooms begin to soften. Add the celery, carrots, and parsnip and stir for 2 minutes. Add the water and the broth and simmer for 45 minutes. Stir in the barley and simmer for 45 minutes longer, or until the barley is soft. Sprinkle with fresh parsley or dill, if using.

Makes 4 main-dish servings (8 cups)

Per serving: 462 calories, 52 g protein, 39 g carbohydrates, 11 g fat, 100 mg cholesterol, 670 mg sodium, 9 g dietary fiber
Diet Exchanges: 2 vegetable, 2 bread, 7 meat, 1 ¹/₂ fat
Carb Choices: 3

CHICKEN AND VEGETABLE SOUP

Prep time: 20 minutes • Cook time: 45 minutes

4   skinless, bone-in chicken breast halves, well trimmed (about 2 pounds)

2   large cloves garlic, minced

1   tablespoon chopped fresh thyme

½   teaspoon salt

¼   teaspoon freshly ground black pepper

5   cups chicken broth

1   cup water

3   medium carrots, cut into chunks (1 ½ cups)

2   medium white turnips, peeled and cut into wedges

3   ribs celery with leaves, cut into 1" pieces

2   medium onions, cut into wedges

½   cup chopped fresh flat-leaf parsley

With kitchen shears, cut the chicken breasts in half crosswise. In a cup, mix the garlic, thyme, ¼ teaspoon of the salt, and the pepper. Rub the mixture all over the chicken and place the chicken in a Dutch oven.

Add the broth, water, carrots, turnips, celery, onions, and the remaining ¼ teaspoon salt. Cover and bring to a boil over high heat. Reduce the heat to low and simmer, covered, for 45 minutes, or until the vegetables are tender and the chicken is no longer pink.

Stir in the parsley and ladle into deep soup bowls.

Makes 4 to 6 main-dish servings (12 cups)

Per serving: 323 calories, 48 g protein, 21 g carbohydrates, 5 g fat, 105 mg cholesterol, 1,490 mg sodium, 5 g dietary fiber
Diet Exchanges: 4 vegetable, 6 meat, ½ fat
Carb Choices: 1

LATIN CHICKEN AND RICE SOUP

Prep time: 20 minutes • Cook time: 47 minutes

$\frac{1}{2}$ cup brown rice

1 pound trimmed boneless, skinless chicken breast halves, cut into 1" chunks

1 tablespoon chili powder

$\frac{1}{2}$ teaspoon salt

$\frac{1}{2}$ teaspoon freshly ground black pepper

2 tablespoons olive oil

2 large onions, halved and cut into thick slices

4 cloves garlic, minced

5 cups chicken broth

4 large carrots, cut into thick slices

1 can (15 $\frac{1}{2}$ ounces) chickpeas, rinsed and drained

1 ripe avocado, halved, pitted, peeled, and cut into chunks

2 teaspoons grated lime peel

$\frac{1}{4}$ cup lime juice

In a heavy medium saucepan, cook the rice according to package directions. Remove from the heat and set aside, covered.

Meanwhile, in a medium bowl, mix the chicken, 1 $\frac{1}{2}$ teaspoons of the chili powder, $\frac{1}{4}$ teaspoon salt, and $\frac{1}{4}$ teaspoon pepper. Cover and set aside.

Heat the oil in a Dutch oven over medium-high heat. Add the onions and garlic and cook, stirring often, for 8 minutes, or until tender and light golden. Stir in the remaining 1 $\frac{1}{2}$ teaspoons chili powder, $\frac{1}{4}$ teaspoon salt, and $\frac{1}{4}$ teaspoon pepper. Cook, stirring, for 1 minute.

Add the broth, carrots, and 2 cups water. Cover and bring to a boil. Reduce the heat to medium and simmer, covered, for 5 minutes, or until the carrots are tender.

Add the chickpeas and chicken. Lower the heat, cover, and simmer, stirring once or twice, for 8 minutes, or until the chicken is no longer pink. Stir in the rice, cover, and cook for 2 minutes longer. Remove from the heat and stir in the avocado, lime peel, and lime juice. Serve immediately.

Note: You can cook the rice a day or so ahead. If not serving the soup right away, or if you're freezing it, leave out the avocado, lime peel, and lime juice. Add them right before serving so their flavors remain fresh.

Makes 6 main-dish servings (14 cups)

Per serving: 333 calories, 25 g protein, 32 g carbohydrates, 12 g fat, 45 mg cholesterol, 1,260 mg sodium, 8 g dietary fiber
Diet Exchanges: 2 vegetable, 1 bread, 3 meat, 2 fat
Carb Choices: 2

WHITE BEAN AND SQUASH SOUP WITH SAUSAGE AND SAGE

Prep time: 40 minutes • **Cook time: 1 hour 25 minutes** • **Stand time: Overnight**

1½ cups Great Northern or navy beans, sorted and rinsed

4 cups water

2 cups chicken broth

8 cloves garlic, peeled

2 sprigs fresh sage + 1 tablespoon chopped

½ teaspoon freshly ground black pepper

2 cups ½" pieces peeled and seeded butternut squash

1 medium leek, halved lengthwise, well washed, and cut into ½" slices

2 ribs celery, sliced

¼ teaspoon salt

1 teaspoon olive oil

2 links (8 ounces) Italian-style sweet or hot turkey sausage, sliced

¼ cup freshly grated Parmesan cheese

Place the beans in a Dutch oven. Add water to cover by 2". Cover and let soak overnight. Drain and rinse and return to the pot.

Add the 4 cups water, the broth, garlic, sage sprigs, and pepper. Cover and bring to a boil over high heat. Reduce the heat to low and simmer, covered, stirring occasionally, for 1 hour, or until the beans are very tender.

Discard the sage sprigs. With a spoon, mash the garlic cloves against the side of the pot.

Add the squash, leek, celery, and salt to the beans, increase the heat, and bring to a boil. Lower the heat, cover, and simmer for 10 minutes.

Meanwhile, in a medium nonstick skillet, heat the oil over medium heat. Add the sausages and cook, turning often, for 5 minutes, or until cooked through. Drain on paper towels.

Add the sausages and chopped sage to the soup. Simmer, uncovered, for 10 minutes, or until the vegetables are tender and the soup is lightly thickened. Ladle into bowls and top with some cheese.

Makes 6 main-dish servings (10 cups)

Per serving: 377 calories, 20 g protein, 42 g carbohydrates, 15 g fat, 30 mg cholesterol, 800 mg sodium, 15 g dietary fiber
Diet Exchanges: 2 vegetable, 2 bread, 2 meat, 2 fat
Carb Choices: 3

CONFETTI CLAM SOUP

Photo on page 95.

Prep time: 30 minutes • Cook time: 45 minutes

4 teaspoons olive oil

1 large onion, chopped

2 ribs celery, coarsely chopped

2 large red and/or yellow bell peppers, coarsely chopped

½ teaspoon freshly ground black pepper

3 ounces Canadian bacon, chopped

3 cloves garlic, minced

4 teaspoons chopped fresh thyme

3 cups chicken broth

12 ounces new potatoes, cut into ½" chunks

1 can (14 ½ ounces) diced tomatoes, drained

½ cup dry white wine (optional)

1½ cups water

2 dozen littleneck clams, well scrubbed

Heat the oil in a Dutch oven over medium heat. Add the onion, celery, bell peppers, and black pepper. Stir well, cover, and cook, stirring occasionally, for 12 to 14 minutes, or until the vegetables are tender.

Stir in the Canadian bacon, garlic, and thyme. Increase the heat to medium-high and cook and stir for 5 minutes, or until all the juices have evaporated.

Add the broth and potatoes, cover, and bring to a boil. Reduce the heat to medium-low and simmer, covered, for 10 minutes, or until the potatoes are tender. Stir in the tomatoes and wine (if using), cover, and simmer for 5 minutes longer. Remove from the heat.

In a covered medium skillet, bring the water to a boil over high heat. Add the clams. Reduce the heat to medium, cover, and cook, stirring often, for 8 to 10 minutes, or until the clams open.

With tongs, transfer the clams to a bowl, discarding those that don't open. Line a fine-mesh strainer with dampened paper towels. Pour the clam broth through the strainer into a glass measure, leaving any sand behind. Add the broth to the soup. Reheat if necessary.

Remove the clams from their shells and chop coarsely. Add the clams to the soup, reheat briefly, and ladle into bowls.

Makes 6 first-course servings (9 ½ cups soup without clams)

Per serving: 169 calories, 14 g protein, 20 g carbohydrates, 5 g fat, 25 mg cholesterol, 770 mg sodium, 4 g dietary fiber
Diet Exchanges: 2 vegetable, 1 ½ meat, 1 fat
Carb Choices: 3

MISO SOUP WITH ASPARAGUS AND BROILED SALMON

Prep time: 20 minutes • Cook time: 25 minutes

4 3-ounce salmon fillets, skinned

2 tablespoons miso paste

1 tablespoon reduced-sodium soy sauce

1 tablespoon canola oil

2 cloves garlic, minced

1½ teaspoons minced peeled fresh ginger

2 tablespoons shao-hsing cooking wine or dry sherry, optional (see note)

3 cups vegetable broth

2 cups ¼" slices bok choy (halve wide stems lengthwise and slice crosswise)

1 cup sugar snap peas, stringed

1 cup 1"-pieces asparagus

2 carrots, cut into matchsticks

½ cup diagonally sliced scallions

Place the salmon in a pie plate. Mix 1 tablespoon of the miso paste and the soy sauce in a cup and spread over the top of the salmon. Set aside.

Preheat the broiler. Line a broiler pan with foil. Coat the broiler-pan rack with cooking spray.

Place the oil, garlic, and ginger in a heavy large saucepan and cook over medium heat, stirring, for 1 to 2 minutes, or until fragrant.

Add the shao-hsing or sherry (if using) and vegetable broth, increase the heat, cover, and bring to a boil. Reduce the heat to medium. Add the bok choy, peas, asparagus, and carrots. Cover and cook for 5 to 6 minutes, or until crisp-tender. Add the scallions and remove from the heat. Stir in the remaining 1 tablespoon miso and cover to keep warm.

After adding the vegetables to the broth, begin to cook the salmon. Broil the salmon 5" from the heat source for 8 to 10 minutes, or until browned and just opaque in the thickest part.

Transfer the salmon to soup bowls, ladle the soup on top, and serve immediately.

Note: Shao-hsing cooking wine is found in any Asian grocery and many large supermarkets. It's also inexpensive.

Makes 4 main-dish servings (4 ¾ cups soup without salmon)

Per serving: 280 calories, 22 g protein, 18 g carbohydrates, 13 g fat, 50 mg cholesterol, 1,120 mg sodium, 4 g dietary fiber
Diet Exchanges: 2 vegetable, ½ bread, 2 ½ meat, 1 fat
Carb Choices: 1

VERY CLASSY BLACK BEAN SOUP

Prep time: 30 minutes • Cook time: 45 minutes

2 tablespoons olive oil

2 large onions, chopped

6 cloves garlic, minced

½ serrano chile pepper, seeded and minced, or 1 jalapeño chile pepper, minced, with the seeds (wear plastic gloves when handling)

3 cans (15 ½ ounces each) black beans, rinsed and drained

4 cups water

½ teaspoon salt

½ teaspoon freshly ground black pepper

2 tablespoons medium-dry sherry (optional)

2 hard-cooked eggs, coarsely chopped

⅓ cup chopped sweet onion

Lemon slices

In a Dutch oven, heat the oil over medium heat. Add the onions, garlic, and chile pepper. Cook, stirring often, for 7 minutes, or until light golden.

Stir in the beans, water, salt, pepper, and sherry (if using). Cover and bring to a boil over high heat. Reduce the heat to low and simmer, covered, for 30 minutes to blend the flavors.

With a potato masher, mash the soup in the pot to a chunky, thick texture.

Ladle the soup into bowls and garnish each with some chopped egg and onion and a lemon slice.

Makes 4 main-dish or 6 first-course servings (7 cups)

Per serving: 200 calories, 8 g protein, 26 g carbohydrates, 9 g fat, 95 mg cholesterol, 680 mg sodium, 7 g dietary fiber
Diet Exchanges: 2 vegetable, 1 bread, ½ meat, 1 ½ fat
Carb Choices: 2

SHAVED BARBECUE BEEF SANDWICHES WITH SPICY SLAW

Photo on page 96.

Prep time: 15 minutes • Cook time: 5 minutes

$^1/_3$ cup smoky barbecue sauce + additional for serving

1 scallion, thinly sliced

12 ounces sliced roast beef, cut into 2" × $^1/_2$" strips

2 tablespoons reduced-fat sour cream

2 tablespoons light mayonnaise

1 tablespoon prepared horseradish

2 teaspoons white wine vinegar

1 teaspoon honey

1 teaspoon jalapeño pepper sauce

3 cups shredded cabbage and carrot coleslaw mix

4 soft whole wheat rolls or sandwich buns

In a small saucepan, bring the barbecue sauce and scallion to a simmer. Stir in the beef and bring to a bare simmer. Cover, remove from the heat, and set aside.

In a medium bowl, stir together the sour cream, mayonnaise, horseradish, vinegar, honey, and pepper sauce until blended. Toss in the coleslaw until evenly coated with the dressing.

Open up the rolls and spoon the beef mixture on the roll bottoms, dividing evenly. Spoon the slaw over the beef, dividing evenly, and cover with the roll tops. Serve with additional barbecue sauce, if you wish.

Makes 4 servings

Per serving: 319 calories, 22 g protein, 42 g carbohydrates, 8 g fat, 45 mg cholesterol, 1,350 mg sodium, 5 g dietary fiber
Diet Exchanges: 1 vegetable, 2 bread, 2 $^1/_2$ meat, 1 fat
Carb Choices: 3

TURKEY PICADILLO SANDWICHES

Prep time: 30 minutes • Cook time: 31 minutes

1 teaspoon olive oil

1 large onion, finely chopped

1 large red bell pepper, chopped

3/4 pound ground turkey breast meat

2 cloves garlic, chopped

1 tablespoon chili powder

2 teaspoons ground cumin

1/4 teaspoon ground cinnamon

1 can (16 ounces) no-salt-added tomato
sauce

3 tablespoons balsamic vinegar

1/3 cup golden raisins, chopped

1/4 cup pimiento-stuffed green olives,
chopped

1/4 teaspoon salt

1/4 teaspoon freshly ground black pepper

4 soft whole wheat sandwich buns

Heat a nonstick skillet over medium heat. Add the oil, onion, and bell pepper and cook for
10 minutes, or until softened, stirring occasionally. Increase the heat to medium-high and add
the turkey. Cook for 5 minutes, or until browned and no longer pink in the center, breaking up the
meat with a spoon.

Stir in the garlic, chili powder, cumin, and cinnamon and cook for 1 minute. Add the tomato sauce,
vinegar, raisins, olives, salt, and black pepper. Bring to a simmer and cook for 15 minutes, or until
thickened, stirring occasionally.

Spoon the meat mixture onto the bottom halves of the buns, dividing evenly. Cover with the bun
tops.

Makes 4 servings

Per serving: 391 calories, 21 g protein, 53 g carbohydrates, 12 g fat, 65 mg cholesterol, 620 mg sodium, 8 g dietary fiber
Diet Exchanges: 1 fruit, 3 vegetable, 2 bread, 2 meat, 1/2 fat
Carb Choices: 4

SICILIAN TUNA ON WHOLE GRAIN BREAD

Prep time: 10 minutes

1 can (6 ounces) solid white tuna in water, drained

3 tablespoons finely chopped carrot

3 tablespoons finely chopped celery

2 tablespoons finely chopped red onion

2 tablespoons finely chopped parsley

2 teaspoons capers, drained

2 ½ teaspoons olive oil

1 ½ teaspoons lemon juice

⅛ teaspoon crushed fennel seeds

⅛ teaspoon salt

⅛ teaspoon freshly ground black pepper

4 slices multigrain bread

In a medium bowl, combine the tuna, carrot, celery, onion, parsley, and capers. Mix well to combine. Stir in the olive oil, lemon juice, fennel seeds, salt, and pepper. Place 2 slices of the bread on a work surface and top each with half of the tuna mixture. Top with the remaining bread slices.

Note: Prepare the tuna and chopped vegetables the day before and refrigerate until ready to use. Before serving, stir in the capers, olive oil, lemon juice, fennel seeds, salt, and pepper.

Makes 2 servings

Per serving: 270 calories, 26 g protein, 29 g carbohydrates, 6 g fat, 35 mg cholesterol, 900 mg sodium, 5 g dietary fiber
Diet Exchanges: ½ vegetable, 2 bread, 3 meat
Carb Choices: 2

CHICKPEA, FLAXSEED, AND OATMEAL BURGERS WITH TZATZIKI

Prep time: 20 minutes • Cook time: 10 minutes

TZATZIKI

½ medium cucumber, peeled, seeded, grated, and squeezed dry

¼ cup fat-free plain yogurt

½ teaspoon minced garlic

⅛ teaspoon salt

⅛ teaspoon freshly ground black pepper

BURGERS

6 tablespoons flaxseed

1 can (15 ½ ounces) chickpeas, rinsed and drained

¼ cup rolled oats

2 cloves garlic

2 tablespoons water

¼ cup chopped fresh mint

2 tablespoons lemon juice

2 teaspoons ground cumin

1 teaspoon salt

⅛ teaspoon freshly ground black pepper

¼ cup panko bread crumbs

1 egg, lightly beaten

1 tablespoon olive oil

4 whole wheat hamburger buns

1 medium tomato, cut into 8 slices

½ cup alfalfa sprouts

To make the tzatziki: In a small bowl, combine the cucumber, yogurt, garlic, salt, and pepper. Cover and refrigerate while preparing the burgers.

To make the burgers: In a spice or coffee grinder, process 5 tablespoons of the flaxseed to a fine meal. In the bowl of a food processor, combine the chickpeas, oats, garlic, and water. Pulse until the mixture is coarsely chopped. Add the mint, lemon juice, cumin, salt, pepper, and flaxseed meal. Pulse the food processor until the mixture is just combined. Divide the mixture into 4 equal portions and shape each into a $1/2$"-thick patty.

Combine the bread crumbs and remaining flaxseed on a plate. Dip the burgers in the egg, then dredge in the bread crumb mixture.

In a large nonstick skillet, heat the oil over medium-high heat. Add the burgers and cook for 5 to 6 minutes per side, or until golden.

On the bottom of each bun, place 2 tomato slices and 2 tablespoons alfalfa sprouts. Place the burgers on top of the sprouts and top each burger with a slightly rounded tablespoon of the tzatziki.

Makes 4 servings

Per serving: 408 calories, 15 g protein, 60 g carbohydrates, 14 g fat, 45 mg cholesterol, 1,220 mg sodium, 13 g dietary fiber
Diet Exchanges: $1/2$ vegetable, 4 bread, $1/2$ meat, 2 fat
Carb Choices: 4

LEMONY SHRIMP AND FENNEL SALAD SANDWICHES

Prep time: 15 minutes

¼ cup low-fat plain yogurt

1½ tablespoons light mayonnaise

1 tablespoon lemon juice

1 teaspoon grated lemon peel

¼ teaspoon sugar

¼ teaspoon salt

⅛ teaspoon hot red-pepper sauce

½ small fennel bulb, cored, trimmed, thinly sliced crosswise, and coarsely chopped into ¾" pieces

8 ounces medium shrimp, cooked

2 tablespoons chopped fennel fronds or parsley

2 tablespoons chopped peeled shallots or scallions

8 slices whole grain bread, toasted

8 soft lettuce leaves

In a medium bowl, whisk together the yogurt, mayonnaise, lemon juice, lemon peel, sugar, salt, and pepper sauce until blended. Add the fennel, shrimp, fennel fronds or parsley, and shallots or scallions to the bowl. Toss to combine.

Set 4 slices of bread on a cutting board. Top each with 2 lettuce leaves. Spoon the salad on top, dividing evenly and spreading level. Top with the remaining bread slices and cut on the diagonal.

Note: The salad can be made up to 6 hours in advance and kept refrigerated.

Makes 4 servings

Per serving: 238 calories, 19 g protein, 32 g carbohydrates, 5 g fat, 115 mg cholesterol, 650 mg sodium, 5 g dietary fiber
Diet Exchanges: ½ vegetable, 2 bread, 2 meat, ½ fat
Carb Choices: 2

FILL-YOU-UP SALADS (REALLY!)

FAST   SUPER FAST   FAST PREP

CURRIED SWEET POTATO SALAD

Photo on page 121.

Prep time: 20 minutes • Cook time: 14 minutes

2 pounds sweet potatoes, peeled and cut into rough ³/₄" chunks

3 tablespoons pecans

¹/₂ cup fat-free plain yogurt

2 tablespoons light mayonnaise

2 tablespoons brown sugar

¹/₂ teaspoon curry powder

¹/₈ teaspoon salt

1 cup juice-packed canned pineapple tidbits, drained

3 scallions, sliced

Place the sweet potatoes in a large saucepan and barely cover with cold water. Cover and bring to a boil over high heat. Reduce the heat to low, and simmer, covered, for 10 to 12 minutes, or until tender. Drain and let cool.

Meanwhile, cook the pecans in a small nonstick skillet over medium heat, stirring often, for 3 to 4 minutes, or until lightly toasted. Tip onto a plate and let cool. Chop coarsely.

In a salad bowl, whisk the yogurt, mayonnaise, sugar, curry powder, and salt until well blended. Add the pineapple, scallions, and sweet potatoes. Mix gently with a rubber spatula. Sprinkle with the toasted pecans and serve immediately, or cover and chill until ready to serve.

Makes 6 side-dish servings

Per serving: 241 calories, 4 g protein, 49 g carbohydrates, 4 g fat, 0 mg cholesterol, 125 mg sodium, 6 g dietary fiber
Diet Exchanges: ¹/₂ fruit, 2 ¹/₂ bread, ¹/₂ fat
Carb Choices: 3

BROCCOLI AND NAPA CABBAGE SALAD
WITH MISO DRESSING

Prep time: 15 minutes • Cook time: 10 minutes

1 tablespoon sesame seeds

2 cups small broccoli florets

1½ tablespoons mellow white miso

1½ tablespoons rice wine vinegar

1 tablespoon canola oil

2 teaspoons reduced-sodium soy sauce

1 teaspoon flax oil

¾ teaspoon finely grated peeled fresh ginger

½ teaspoon brown sugar

4 cups sliced napa cabbage or iceberg lettuce (1"-thick slices)

½ cup thinly sliced radishes

1 kirby cucumber, thinly sliced

2 scallions, thinly sliced

1 large carrot, peeled

In a small skillet, cook the sesame seeds over medium heat, tossing, for 2 minutes, until light golden. Tip out onto a plate and let cool.

Bring ½" water to a boil in a medium saucepan. Add the broccoli, cover, and cook, stirring several times, for 4 minutes, until crisp-tender. Drain and cool briefly under cold running water.

In a salad bowl, whisk together the miso, rice vinegar, canola oil, soy sauce, flax oil, ginger, and sugar, until well blended.

Add the cabbage or lettuce, radishes, cucumber, scallions, and broccoli. With a vegetable peeler, peel long, curly strands from the carrot, letting them drop into the salad bowl. Toss the salad to mix, sprinkle with the toasted sesame seeds, and serve.

Makes 4 side-dish servings

Per serving: 110 calories, 4 g protein, 12 g carbohydrates, 6 g fat, 0 mg cholesterol, 330 mg sodium, 5 g dietary fiber
Diet Exchanges: 2 vegetable, 1 fat
Carb Choices: 1

CANTALOUPE AND WATERCRESS SALAD WITH PICKLED ONIONS

Photo on page 122.

Prep time: 20 minutes

⅓ cup coarsely chopped red onion

¼ teaspoon grated lime peel

2 tablespoons lime juice

⅛ teaspoon salt

1 tablespoon olive oil

2 tablespoons honey

¼ teaspoon freshly ground black pepper

3 cups ¾" chunks ripe cantaloupe

2 ripe plums, thinly sliced

1 bunch watercress, tough stems trimmed

2 tablespoons crumbled goat cheese or feta cheese

2 tablespoons sliced almonds or pumpkin seeds

In a salad bowl, mix the onion, lime peel, lime juice, salt, oil, honey, and pepper with a fork. Stir to combine.

Add the cantaloupe, plums, watercress, cheese, and almonds or pumpkin seeds, and toss to mix. Serve immediately.

Makes 6 first-course servings

Per serving: 110 calories, 2 g protein, 18 g carbohydrates, 4 g fat, 0 mg cholesterol, 75 mg sodium, 2 g dietary fiber
Diet Exchanges: 1 fruit, 1 fat
Carb Choices: 1

GRAPEFRUIT, MANGO, AND AVOCADO SALAD
WITH SHERRY DRESSING

Prep time: 20 minutes

1 tablespoon olive oil	1 large pink grapefruit
1 tablespoon medium-dry sherry or sherry vinegar	4 cups colorful mixed baby greens
1 ½ teaspoons red wine vinegar	1 cup sliced ripe avocado
¼ teaspoon salt	1 cup sliced ripe mango
⅛ teaspoon freshly ground black pepper	2 tablespoons chopped red onion

In a salad bowl, mix the oil, sherry or sherry vinegar, red wine vinegar, salt, and pepper with a fork.

With a serrated knife, peel the grapefruit, cutting off most, but not all, of the white pith. Working over a bowl, cut out the fruit from between the membranes. Add 1 ½ tablespoons of the grapefruit juice to the dressing and mix well.

Add the greens, avocado, mango, red onion, and the grapefruit sections to the dressing and toss gently to mix. Serve immediately.

Makes 4 first-course servings

Per serving: 129 calories, 2 g protein, 12 g carbohydrates, 9 g fat, 0 mg cholesterol, 220 mg sodium, 4 g dietary fiber
Diet Exchanges: ½ fruit, ½ vegetable, 2 fat
Carb Choices: 1

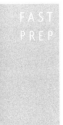

PINEAPPLE AND STRAWBERRIES
WITH CILANTRO AND PEPPER

Photo on page 123.

Prep time: 10 minutes • **Stand time: 15 minutes** • **Chill time: 30 minutes**

2 **cups hulled and quartered fresh strawberries**

1 **tablespoon packed brown sugar**

4 **cups ½" chunks fresh pineapple**

¼ **cup chopped fresh cilantro**

¼ **teaspoon ground cinnamon**

⅛ **teaspoon ground cumin**

¼ **teaspoon freshly ground black pepper**

Mix the strawberries and sugar in a serving bowl. Let stand for 15 minutes to let the juices flow.

Add the pineapple, cilantro, cinnamon, cumin, and pepper to the strawberries and stir gently to mix. Cover and chill for at least 30 minutes, or until ready to serve.

Makes 6 to 8 side-dish servings

Per serving: 75 calories, 1 g protein, 19 g carbohydrates, 1 g fat, 0 mg cholesterol, 0 mg sodium, 3 g dietary fiber
Diet Exchanges: 1 fruit
Carb Choices: 1

SPINACH AND STRAWBERRY SALAD WITH FRESH MOZZARELLA

FAST

Prep time: 18 minutes • Cook time: 5 minutes

3 **tablespoons chopped whole or slivered almonds**

2 **cups hulled and sliced strawberries**

2 **tablespoons extra-virgin olive oil**

2 **tablespoons honey**

1 **tablespoon + 1 teaspoon balsamic vinegar**

½ **teaspoon salt**

⅛ **teaspoon freshly ground black pepper**

1 **bag (6 ounces) baby spinach**

1 **ripe medium mango, peeled and cut in small chunks**

3 **small balls fresh mozzarella (about 5 ounces total), cut in small chunks**

1 **ripe avocado, peeled and cut in small chunks**

Cook the almonds in a small skillet over medium heat, tossing often, for 3 to 4 minutes, or until lightly toasted. Tip onto a plate and let cool.

Put ½ cup of the strawberries, the oil, honey, and balsamic vinegar in a food processor. Process until smooth. Scrape into a salad bowl and stir in the salt and pepper.

Add the spinach, mango, the toasted almonds, and the remaining 1½ cups strawberries to the dressing and toss to mix well. Sprinkle the mozzarella and avocado over the top.

Makes 4 main-dish servings

Per serving: 330 calories, 10 g protein, 26 g carbohydrates, 22 g fat, 30 mg cholesterol, 420 mg sodium, 6 g dietary fiber
Diet Exchanges: ½ fruit, 1 vegetable, ½ bread, 1 meat, 4 fat
Carb Choices: 2

SPRING'S BEST SALAD

Prep time: 15 minutes • **Cook time: 26 minutes**

3 **large eggs**	½ **cup sliced radishes**
½ **pound small thin-skinned potatoes, scrubbed and quartered**	½ **cup halved grape tomatoes**
2 **pinches of salt**	1 **knobby spring onion, or 3 scallions, thinly sliced**
1 **pound asparagus, tough stems trimmed, cut into 2" lengths**	⅓ **cup Herbed Mustard Vinaigrette (page 86) or Roasted Garlic Vinaigrette (page 87)**
4 **cups baby spinach**	**Freshly ground black pepper**

Place the eggs in a small saucepan and cover with cold water. Bring to a boil over high heat. Reduce the heat to low and simmer slowly for 10 minutes. Cool under cold running water and shell.

Place the potatoes in a medium saucepan and add a pinch of salt. Barely cover with cold water, cover, and bring to a boil over high heat. Reduce the heat to medium and cook for 8 to 10 minutes, or until tender. Drain and cool briefly under cold running water.

Place 1" of water in the same medium saucepan and bring to a boil over high heat. Add a pinch of salt and the asparagus and cook, stirring often, for 3 to 4 minutes, or until bright green and crisp-tender. Drain and cool briefly under cold running water.

On a large platter, make a bed of the spinach. Cut the eggs into wedges. Place the eggs, potatoes, asparagus, radishes, and tomatoes in mounds. Sprinkle with the onion. Spoon the dressing over or serve on the side. Season to taste with the pepper.

Note: For a little more variety, try adding 1 can of flaked water-packed tuna, salmon, or some cooked and shelled medium shrimp.

Makes 4 main-dish servings

Per serving: 207 calories, 11 g protein, 21 g carbohydrates, 10 g fat, 160 mg cholesterol, 250 mg sodium, 6 g dietary fiber
Diet Exchanges: 2 vegetable, ½ bread, 1 meat, 1 ½ fat
Carb Choices: 1

CHICKEN AND ASPARAGUS SALAD
WITH TARRAGON DRESSING

Prep time: 12 minutes • Cook time: 30 minutes

2 boneless, skinless chicken breast halves (6 ounces each)

Pinch of salt

2 large eggs

1 pound asparagus, tough ends trimmed, cut into 1" pieces

$\frac{1}{4}$ cup + 2 tablespoons light mayonnaise

1 teaspoon grated lemon zest

1 tablespoon lemon juice

$\frac{1}{2}$ teaspoon dried tarragon, crumbled

$\frac{1}{2}$ teaspoon grainy mustard

$\frac{1}{2}$ teaspoon freshly ground black pepper

1 cup roughly chopped cucumber

1 cup thinly sliced celery

4 scallions, thinly sliced

2 tablespoons coarsely chopped walnuts

Place the chicken breasts in a medium skillet. Add water to just cover and salt. Cover and bring to a boil over high heat. Reduce the heat to low and simmer slowly, turning the chicken once, for 8 to 10 minutes, until cooked through. Transfer to a plate and let stand until cool enough to handle. Tear into pieces.

Meanwhile, place the eggs in a medium saucepan and cover with cold water. Bring to a boil over high heat. Reduce the heat to low and simmer slowly for 10 minutes. Cool under cold running water and shell. Remove the yolks and save for another use. Coarsely chop the whites.

In the same saucepan, bring $\frac{1}{2}$" water to a boil over high heat. Add the asparagus and cook, stirring often, for 4 to 5 minutes, until crisp-tender. Drain and cool briefly under cold running water.

In a salad bowl, whisk the mayonnaise, lemon zest and juice, tarragon, mustard, pepper, and $\frac{1}{2}$ teaspoon salt. Add the cucumber, celery, scallions, chicken, egg whites, and asparagus and mix gently with a rubber spatula. Sprinkle with the walnuts and serve.

Makes 4 main-dish servings

Per serving: 260 calories, 26 g protein, 9 g carbohydrates, 14 g fat, 165 mg cholesterol, 310 mg sodium, 3 g dietary fiber
Diet Exchanges: 1 vegetable, 3 $\frac{1}{2}$ meat, 2 fat
Carb Choices: $\frac{1}{2}$

PORK AND CORN SALAD WITH TOMATO-BASIL DRESSING

Prep time: 15 minutes • Cook time: 8 minutes

1 pork tenderloin (12 ounces), well trimmed, cut into $1/2$"- thick slices, each slice halved crosswise

$1/2$ cup slivered fresh basil

2 tablespoons olive oil

2 cloves garlic, minced

$1/2$ teaspoon coarsely ground black pepper

$1/2$ teaspoon salt

6 ounces diced canned tomatoes

2 teaspoons red wine vinegar

$1 1/2$ cups frozen corn kernels

2 cups chopped red bell pepper

3 tablespoons water

4 cups colorful mixed baby greens

Place the pork in a medium bowl. Add $1/4$ cup of the basil, 1 tablespoon of the oil, the garlic, pepper, and $1/4$ teaspoon of the salt. Toss to coat the pork well. Set aside while preparing the rest of the salad.

Place the diced tomatoes in a large salad bowl. Stir in the vinegar and the remaining $1/4$ cup basil, 1 tablespoon oil, and $1/4$ teaspoon salt.

Place the corn, bell pepper, and water in a large nonstick skillet. Cover and cook over medium-high heat, stirring often, for 3 to 4 minutes, or until the corn is tender. Stir into the tomato mixture.

Dry the skillet. Place the pork in the same skillet and cook over medium heat, turning often, for 5 minutes, or until just slightly pink in the thickest part.

Add the pork and any pan juices to the tomato-corn mixture. Add the mixed greens and toss to blend the ingredients and wilt the greens slightly. Serve immediately.

Makes 4 main-dish servings

Per serving: 258 calories, 22 g protein, 23 g carbohydrates, 10 g fat, 55 mg cholesterol, 460 mg sodium, 5 g dietary fiber
Diet Exchanges: 1 vegetable, 1 bread, 3 meat, 2 fat
Carb Choices: 2

CURRIED COUSCOUS SALAD

Prep time: 15 minutes • Cook time: 8 minutes • Stand time: 1 hour

1¼ cups reduced-sodium chicken or vegetable broth

1 small zucchini, coarsely chopped

1–2 teaspoons green curry paste

¼ teaspoon freshly ground black pepper

1 cup whole wheat couscous

⅓ cup chopped dried apricots

3 tablespoons golden raisins

3 tablespoons slivered almonds

1 can (15–16 ounces) small pink beans, chili beans, or red kidney beans, rinsed and drained

1 large tomato, chopped

½ cup coarsely chopped fresh flat-leaf parsley

¼ cup chopped red onion

¼ cup lime juice

2 tablespoons olive oil

Stir the broth, zucchini, curry paste, and pepper in a medium saucepan. Cover and bring to a boil over high heat. Stir in the couscous, apricots, and raisins. Remove from the heat and let stand, covered, for 10 minutes.

Meanwhile, cook the almonds in a small nonstick skillet over medium heat, stirring often, for 3 to 4 minutes, or until lightly toasted. Tip onto a plate and let cool.

Fluff the couscous with a fork. Transfer to a large bowl, cover with a sheet of waxed paper, and let stand for 20 minutes, until cooled.

Add the beans, tomato, parsley, red onion, lime juice, and oil to the couscous mixture and stir to blend well. Cover and let stand for 30 minutes or refrigerate until ready to serve. Sprinkle with the almonds just before serving.

Makes 4 main-dish servings, 6 to 8 side-dish servings

Per serving: 350 calories, 12 g protein, 57 g carbohydrates, 10 g fat, 0 mg cholesterol, 480 mg sodium, 11 g dietary fiber
Diet Exchanges: 2 bread, ½ meat, 2 fat
Carb Choices: 4

MIDDLE-EASTERN SALAD WITH CRISP PITA WEDGES

Prep time: 20 minutes • Cook time: 12 minutes • Cooling time: 10 minutes

2 medium whole wheat pitas (6" diameter)

³⁄₄ teaspoon dried oregano, crumbled

3 tablespoons pine nuts

1 tablespoon sesame seeds

¼ cup lemon juice

3 tablespoons extra-virgin olive oil

1 clove garlic, minced

½ teaspoon paprika

½ teaspoon salt

1 can (15 ounces) pink beans or pinto beans, rinsed and drained

4 scallions, sliced

4 cups sliced romaine lettuce

1 cup chopped red bell pepper

1 cup small radishes, quartered

1 cup cucumber chunks

¼ cup snipped fresh dill

Preheat the oven to 400°F.

With kitchen scissors, cut around the perimeter of each pita to make 2 rounds. Place the rounds rough side up on a baking sheet and sprinkle with ½ teaspoon of the oregano. Place the pine nuts and sesame seeds in a small baking pan or ovenproof skillet.

Bake the pita for 8 to 10 minutes, without turning, until crisp and toasted. Bake the pine nuts and sesame seeds for 4 to 5 minutes, stirring twice, until browned. Remove both from the oven. Leave the pita breads on the baking sheet. Tip the nuts and seeds into a bowl. Let both cool. When the pita is cooled, break into rough 1" chunks.

Meanwhile, in a large salad bowl, mix the lemon juice, oil, garlic, paprika, salt, and the remaining ¼ teaspoon oregano with a fork. Add the beans and scallions, and stir to mix well. Let stand 10 minutes to blend the flavors.

Add the romaine, bell pepper, radishes, cucumber, and dill to the beans. Toss to mix well. Add the toasted pitas, pine nuts, and sesame seeds, and toss again.

Makes 4 main-dish servings

Per serving: 340 calories, 10 g protein, 40 g carbohydrates, 16 g fat, 0 mg cholesterol, 710 mg sodium, 10 g dietary fiber
Diet Exchanges: ½ vegetable, 2 bread, 3 fat
Carb Choices: 3

WARM CHICKEN AND CASHEW STIR-FRY SALAD

Prep time: 25 minutes • Cook time: 14 minutes

12 ounces boneless, skinless chicken breast halves, cut into thin crosswise strips

4 tablespoons reduced-sodium soy sauce

¼–½ teaspoon crushed red-pepper flakes

3 tablespoons raw cashews

2 tablespoons olive or canola oil

5 cloves garlic, slivered

1½ tablespoons slivered peeled fresh ginger

1 large red bell pepper, cut into thin strips

2 medium carrots, cut into thin slices

4 scallions, diagonally sliced

½ cup orange juice

3 cups shredded iceberg lettuce

3 cups baby spinach

In a medium bowl, mix the chicken, 2 tablespoons of the soy sauce, and the red-pepper flakes, to taste. Cover and set aside.

Cook the cashews in a small nonstick skillet over medium heat, stirring often, for 3 to 4 minutes, or until lightly toasted. Tip onto a plate and let cool.

Heat 1 tablespoon of the oil in a large nonstick skillet over medium-high heat. Add the garlic and ginger and stir-fry for 1 to 2 minutes, or until fragrant and lightly golden. Add the chicken and stir-fry for 3 to 4 minutes, or until no longer pink. Transfer to a clean bowl.

Place the remaining 1 tablespoon oil in the same skillet and heat over medium-high heat. Add the bell pepper and carrots, and stir-fry for 3 minutes. Add the scallions and stir-fry for 2 minutes longer, or until the vegetables are crisp-tender. Return the chicken and any juices to the skillet. Add the orange juice and the remaining 2 tablespoons soy sauce. Bring to a boil, stirring. Let boil for 30 seconds; remove from the heat.

Mix the lettuce and spinach on a large, deep platter or in a wide, shallow bowl. Spoon the chicken mixture on top. Sprinkle with the cashews and serve immediately.

Makes 4 main-dish servings

Per serving: 286 calories, 24 g protein, 18 g carbohydrates, 11 g fat, 50 mg cholesterol, 670 mg sodium, 4 g dietary fiber
Diet Exchanges: 2 vegetable, 3 meat, 2 fat
Carb Choices: 1

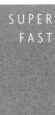

HERBED MUSTARD VINAIGRETTE

This is a good basic dressing that's delicious on mixed greens, steamed asparagus, and boiled potatoes. Change the flavor by adding minced shallot or garlic or substituting lemon juice for the vinegar.

Prep time: 8 minutes

¼ **cup vegetable broth**

2 **tablespoons chopped fresh parsley**

2 **tablespoons red wine vinegar**

4 **teaspoons Dijon mustard**

1½ **teaspoons chopped fresh thyme**

¼ **teaspoon salt**

⅛ **teaspoon freshly ground black pepper**

⅓ **cup olive oil**

Place the broth, parsley, vinegar, mustard, thyme, salt, and pepper in a medium bowl. Whisk until well blended. Whisk in the oil in a slow, steady stream. Transfer to a small jar and refrigerate until ready to serve.

Note: This dressing will keep for 4 to 5 days in the refrigerator.

Makes twelve 1-tablespoon servings (¾ cup)

Per serving: 59 calories, 0 g protein, 0 g carbohydrates, 6 g fat, 0 mg cholesterol, 100 mg sodium, 0 g dietary fiber
Diet Exchanges: 1 fat
Carb Choices: 0

ROASTED GARLIC VINAIGRETTE

Try this vinaigrette on Spring's Best Salad (page 80) or with arugula tossed with sliced ripe pears, toasted pecans, and goat cheese.

Prep time: 12 minutes • Cook time: 45 minutes

1 **medium head garlic, roasted**	½ **teaspoon salt**
3 **tablespoons chicken or vegetable broth**	¼ **teaspoon freshly ground black pepper**
2 **tablespoons balsamic vinegar**	⅓ **cup olive oil**
¼ **cup chopped fresh flat-leaf parsley**	
2 **teaspoons chopped fresh rosemary (optional)**	

Preheat the oven to 400°F.

Cut a thin slice from the top of the garlic to expose the cloves. Place the head cut side up on a large piece of foil. Seal the top and sides of the foil tightly. Place in the oven and roast for 45 to 60 minutes, or until the cloves are very soft and lightly browned. Remove from the oven, open the packet, and set aside until cool enough to handle.

Squeeze the cloves into a medium bowl. With the back of a large metal spoon, mash the garlic to a smooth paste.

Gradually whisk in the broth and vinegar. Whisk in the parsley, rosemary (if using), salt, and pepper. Then whisk in the oil in a slow, steady stream. Transfer to a small jar and refrigerate until ready to serve.

Note: The dressing thickens in the fridge. Let it come to room temperature before using.

Makes twelve 1-tablespoon servings (¾ cup)

Per serving: 64 calories, 0 g protein, 2 g carbohydrates, 6 g fat, 0 mg cholesterol, 115 mg sodium, 0 g dietary fiber
Diet Exchanges: 1 fat
Carb Choices: 0

A FEW LESS THAN A THOUSAND ISLANDS DRESSING

Prep time: 5 minutes

½ **cup light mayonnaise**

¼ **cup fat-free sour cream**

¼ **cup medium-spicy chunky salsa**

2 **tablespoons dill pickle relish**

2 **tablespoons balsamic vinegar**

1 **tablespoon tomato paste**

⅛ **teaspoon salt**

⅛ **teaspoon freshly ground black pepper**

Place the mayonnaise, sour cream, salsa, relish, vinegar, tomato paste, salt, and pepper in a medium bowl. Whisk until blended. Transfer to a small jar and refrigerate until ready to serve.

Makes sixteen 1-tablespoon servings (1 cup)

Per serving: 24 calories, 0 g protein, 3 g carbohydrates, 1 g fat, 0 mg cholesterol, 105 mg sodium, 0 g dietary fiber
Diet Exchanges: 0
Carb Choices: 0

LEMONY YOGURT DRESSING

Prep time: 7 minutes

⅔ **cup fat-free plain yogurt**

3 **tablespoons olive oil**

½ **teaspoon grated lemon peel**

3 **tablespoons lemon juice**

1 **tablespoon chopped fresh mint**

1 **tablespoon chopped fresh cilantro**

1 **teaspoon honey**

¼ **teaspoon dried oregano, crumbled**

½ **teaspoon salt**

⅛ **teaspoon freshly ground black pepper**

Place the yogurt, oil, lemon peel, lemon juice, mint, cilantro, honey, oregano, salt, and pepper in a medium bowl. Whisk until blended. Transfer to a small jar and refrigerate until ready to serve.

Makes eight 2-tablespoon servings (1 cup)

Per serving: 60 calories, 1 g protein, 3 g carbohydrates, 5 g fat, 0 mg cholesterol, 160 mg sodium, 0 g dietary fiber
Diet Exchanges: 1 fat
Carb Choices: 0

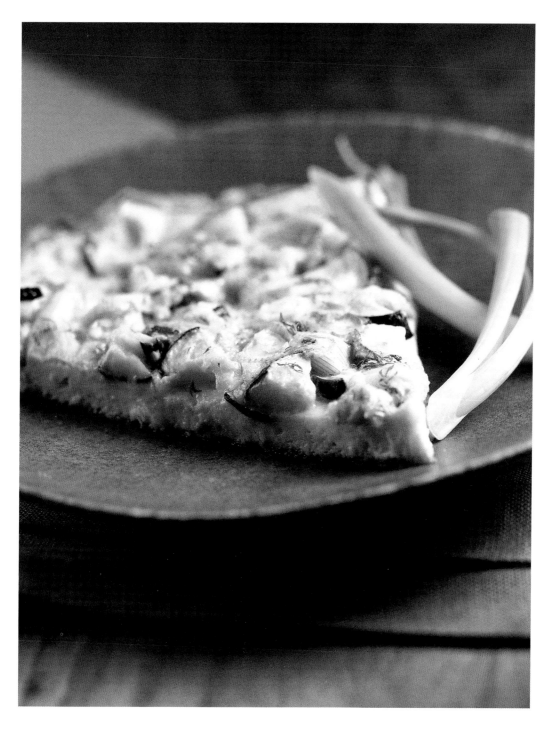

ZUCCHINI AND DILL FRITTATA

Recipe on page 43

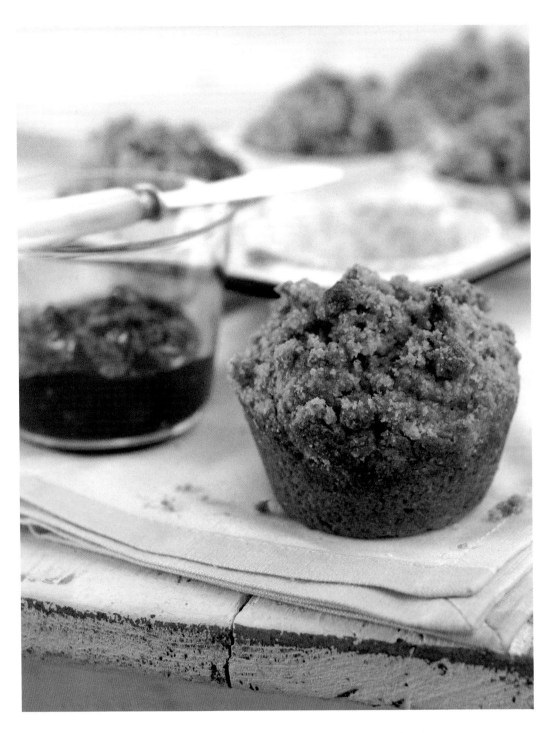

PEANUT BUTTER AND BANANA STREUSEL MUFFINS

Recipe on page 46

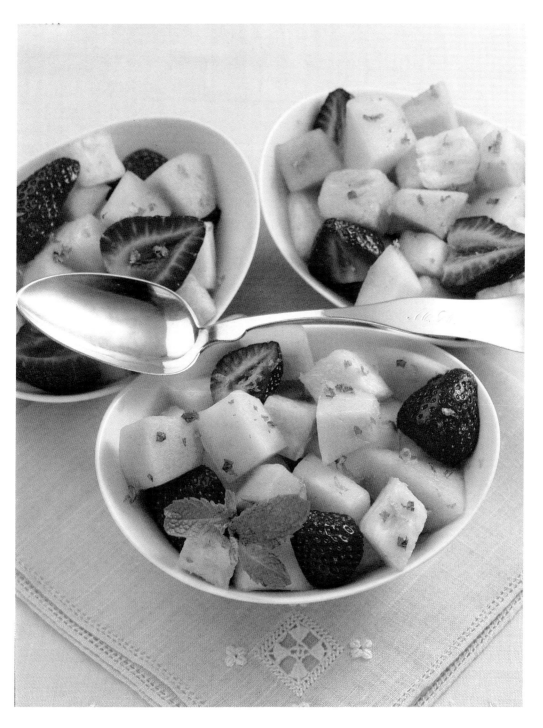

MINTED HONEY-LIME FRUIT SALAD

Recipe on page 48

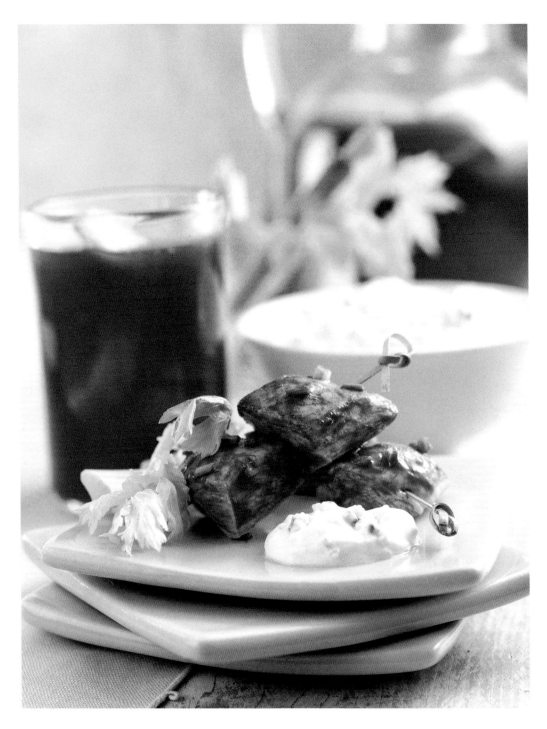

BUFFALO CHICKEN BITES

Recipe on page 52

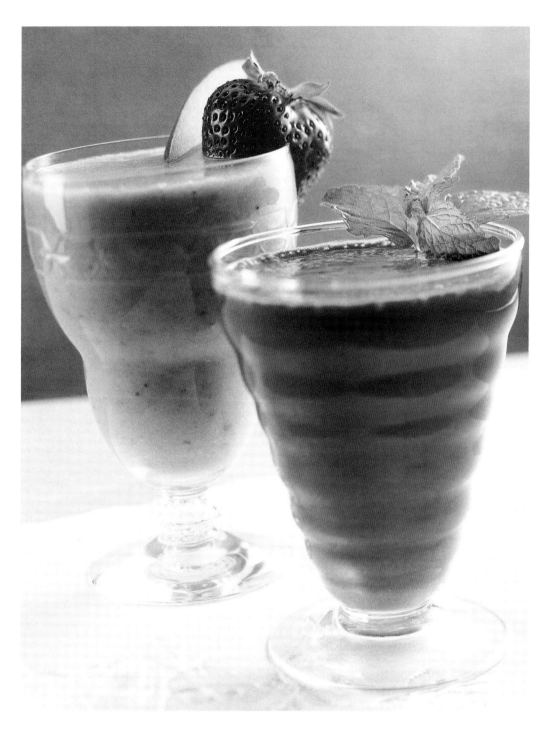

CHOCOLATE MALTED MILKSHAKE AND STRAWBERRY-MANGO SMOOTHIE

Recipe on page 53

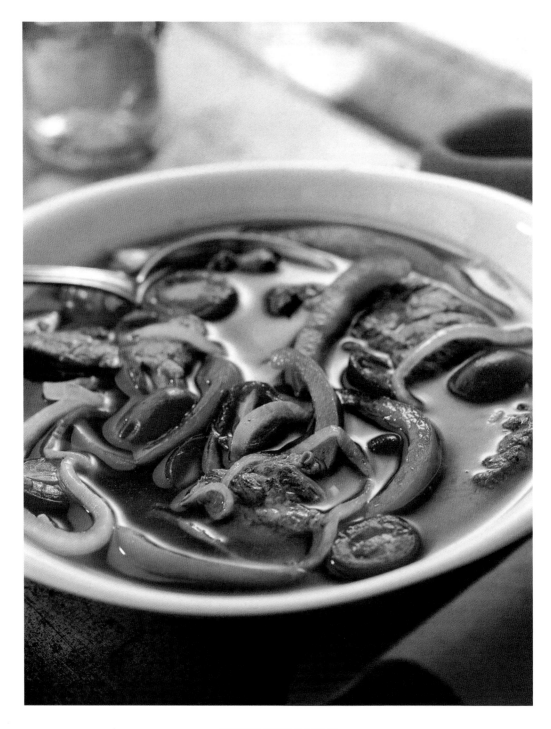

PEPPER STEAK SOUP

Recipe on page 59

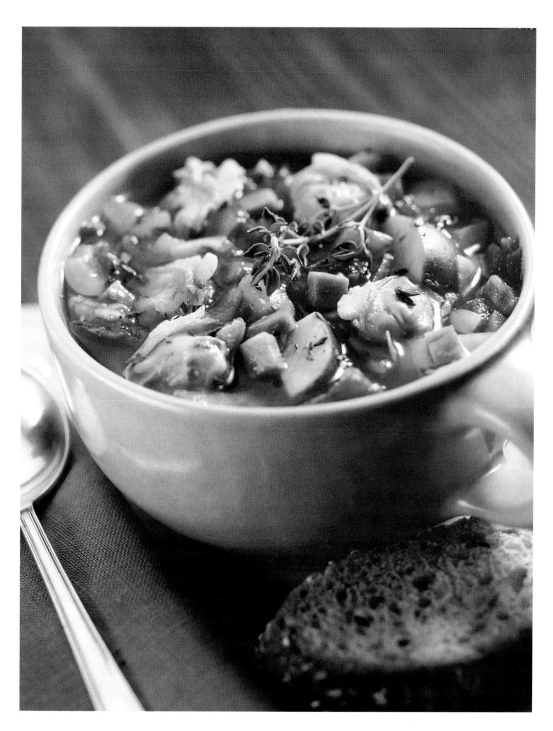

CONFETTI CLAM SOUP

Recipe on page 64

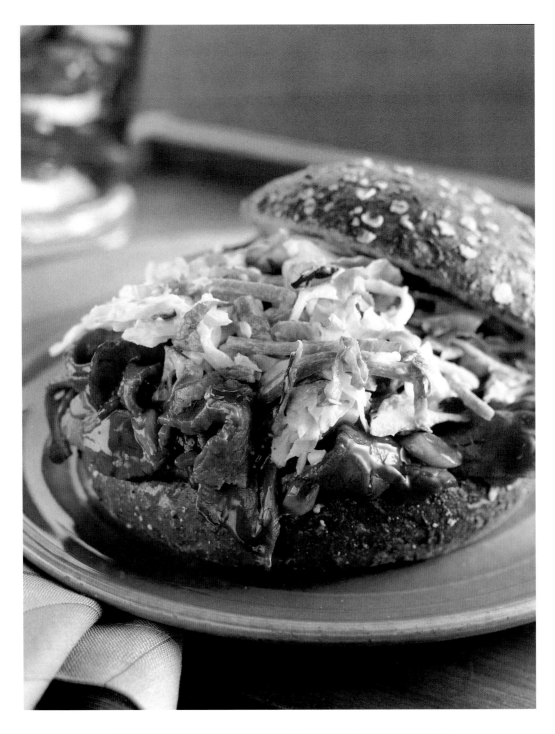

SHAVED BARBECUE BEEF SANDWICHES WITH SPICY SLAW

Recipe on page 67

SIDE DISHES

FAST   SUPER FAST   FAST PREP

ANISE-SCENTED BALSAMIC BEETS

Photo on page 124.

Prep time: 15 minutes • Cook time: 45 minutes • Stand time: 30 minutes

1 **pound beets (about 1 bunch), about 2" in diameter each, trimmed**

1 **cup orange juice**

2 **tablespoons balsamic vinegar**

2 **star anise pods**

1 **tablespoon sugar**

1 **medium bunch arugula (about 4 cups), trimmed and washed**

1 **tablespoon lemon juice**

1 **teaspoon grated lemon zest**

1 **tablespoon olive oil**

¼ **teaspoon salt**

⅛ **teaspoon freshly ground black pepper**

Preheat the oven to 425°F.

Wrap the beets in aluminum foil and place directly on the oven rack. Roast for 45 minutes, or until a knife easily pierces the beets. Cool for 30 minutes, then peel and cut each beet into 8 wedges.

Meanwhile, in a medium saucepan over medium-high heat, combine the orange juice, vinegar, star anise, and sugar. Bring the mixture to a boil and cook for 12 to 14 minutes, or until reduced to about 2 ½ to 3 tablespoons of syrup. Discard the star anise pods, then toss the syrup with the beets.

Toss the arugula with the lemon juice, lemon zest, oil, salt, and pepper. Arrange over 4 serving plates. Divide the beets into 4 portions and place each on top of the arugula. Drizzle any remaining orange-balsamic syrup over each plate. Serve immediately.

Note: The beets and glaze in this recipe can be made up to 3 days in advance. Toss them, chilled, right before serving for a cool salad.

Makes 4 servings

Per serving: 130 calories, 3 g protein, 23 g carbohydrates, 4 g fat, 0 mg cholesterol, 240 mg sodium, 4 g dietary fiber
Diet Exchanges: ½ fruit, 2 vegetable, 1 fat
Carb Choices: 1

CORN ON THE COB WITH CHILE-MAPLE GLAZE

Prep time: 10 minutes ● **Cook time: 25 minutes**

⅓ cup maple syrup

2 tablespoons butter

2 teaspoons lime juice

1 small chipotle chile pepper in adobo sauce, finely minced, about 1 teaspoon (see note)

1 teaspoon reduced-sodium soy sauce

¼ teaspoon ground cumin

¼ teaspoon salt

4 ears corn on the cob, husked

1 tablespoon chopped fresh cilantro (optional)

Coat a grill rack with cooking spray. Preheat the grill.

In a medium saucepan, combine the maple syrup, butter, lime juice, pepper, soy sauce, cumin, and salt. Bring to a simmer over low heat and cook for 12 to 14 minutes, or until thick and syrupy.

Place the corn on the grill rack and grill for 2 minutes. Brush the corn with some of the syrup mixture and turn a quarter turn. Continue brushing and turning the corn every 2 minutes for 6 to 8 minutes longer, or until the corn is well marked and cooked through. Transfer the corn to a serving platter and brush with the remaining syrup. Sprinkle with the cilantro, if using, and serve immediately.

Note: Chile oil sticks to the skin, and water alone won't wash it away. After handling chiles, be sure to use soap and water to wash your hands.

Makes 4 servings

Per serving: 206 calories, 3 g protein, 38 g carbohydrates, 7 g fat, 15 mg cholesterol, 260 mg sodium, 2 g dietary fiber
Diet Exchanges: 2 ½ bread, 1 fat
Carb Choices: 3

SAUTÉED STRING BEANS, SWEET ONION, AND GRAPE TOMATOES

Prep time: 15 minutes • Cook time: 20 minutes

¾ **pound fresh green beans, trimmed and cut in half**

1 **tablespoon olive oil**

1 **small sweet onion, thinly sliced**

1 **red bell pepper, seeded and cut into strips**

2 **cloves garlic, cut into thin slivers**

¼ **teaspoon salt**

⅛ **teaspoon freshly ground black pepper**

1 **pint grape tomatoes, halved**

1 **tablespoon vegetable broth or chicken broth, or water**

2 **teaspoons coarsely chopped fresh marjoram or flat-leaf parsley**

In a large deep skillet, bring ½" water to a boil over high heat. Add the green beans, cover, and cook for 6 to 8 minutes, until tender. Drain.

Dry the skillet. Heat the oil in the same skillet over medium heat. Stir in the onion, bell pepper, garlic, salt, and black pepper. Cook for 6 minutes, stirring often, until tender. Add the tomatoes. Toss well and add the broth or water. Cook for 2 to 3 minutes, stirring often, until the tomatoes start to collapse.

Add the beans and the marjoram or parsley. Toss for 1 minute, until heated through. Serve hot or at room temperature.

Makes 4 servings

Per serving: 90 calories, 2 g protein, 12 g carbohydrates, 3 ½ g fat, 0 mg cholesterol, 90 mg sodium, 5 g dietary fiber
Diet Exchanges: 2 vegetable, 1 fat
Carb Choices: 1

WILD MUSHROOM SAUTÉ

Prep time: 15 minutes • Cook time: 14 minutes

1 tablespoon olive oil

½ cup chopped onion

1 package (10 ounces) sliced white mushrooms (see note)

8 ounces shiitake mushrooms, stemmed and halved

6 ounces oyster mushrooms, trimmed and halved

1 teaspoon chopped fresh rosemary

1 tablespoon minced garlic

½ teaspoon salt

⅛ teaspoon freshly ground black pepper

¼ cup Madeira wine or beef broth

Heat the oil in a large nonstick skillet over medium-high heat. Add the onion and cook for 1 minute. Add the mushrooms and rosemary, mounding them in the skillet. Cook for 10 to 12 minutes, stirring occasionally, until the mushrooms give off their liquid and begin to brown. Add the garlic, salt, and pepper and cook for 2 to 3 minutes longer, or until the garlic begins to brown. Pour in the wine or broth and cook for 1 to 2 minutes, or until the liquid evaporates.

Note: Instead of buying separate types of mushrooms, you can use 4 or 5 packages of mixed wild or domestic mushrooms. This dish can be served with beef, chicken, or cooked pasta.

Makes 4 servings

Per serving: 115 calories, 6 g protein, 12 g carbohydrates, 3 g fat, 0 mg cholesterol, 310 mg sodium, 3 g dietary fiber
Diet Exchanges: 2 vegetable, 1 fat
Carb Choices: 1

HONEY-BAKED ACORN SQUASH

Prep time: 5 minutes • Cook time: 1 hour 15 minutes

1 **acorn squash, about 1 ½ pounds**	**Pinch of freshly ground black pepper**
¼ **teaspoon ground cinnamon**	1 **teaspoon olive oil**
¼ **teaspoon salt**	1 **tablespoon honey**

Preheat the oven to 350°F.

Cut the squash in half and scoop out the seeds. Cut each half in half again and place in a 13" × 9" baking dish.

Sprinkle the cinnamon, salt, and pepper over each squash quarter. Drizzle with the oil and then the honey.

Bake for 1 hour 15 minutes to 1 hour 30 minutes, until the squash is lightly golden and tender when pierced with a fork.

Makes 4 servings

Per serving: 80 calories, 1 g protein, 18 g carbohydrates, 1 ½ g fat, 0 mg cholesterol, 75 mg sodium, 2 g dietary fiber
Diet Exchanges: 2 vegetable
Carb Choices: 1

GLAZED TURNIPS, PEARL ONIONS, AND CARROTS

Photo on page 125.

Photo on page 125.

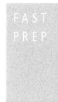

Prep time: 15 minutes • Cook time: 30 minutes

4 peeled turnips (³⁄₄ pound), cut into
   8 wedges each

2 cups frozen small white onions (about
   10 ounces), thawed

1 cup baby carrots

1¹⁄₄ cups chicken broth

2 tablespoons balsamic vinegar

2 tablespoons packed brown sugar

4 teaspoons butter

¹⁄₂ teaspoon ground cumin

¹⁄₄ teaspoon salt

¹⁄₈ teaspoon freshly ground black pepper

2 tablespoons chopped fresh parsley

In a large skillet over medium-high heat, combine the turnips, onions, carrots, broth, vinegar, sugar, butter, cumin, salt, and pepper. Bring to a boil, reduce the heat to medium, and simmer, stirring occasionally, for 20 to 25 minutes, or until the liquid evaporates. Continue cooking, stirring often, for 4 to 6 minutes longer, or until the vegetables are golden and shiny. Remove from the heat and stir in the parsley.

Makes 4 servings

Per serving: 173 calories, 4 g protein, 31 g carbohydrates, 5 g fat, 10 mg cholesterol, 580 mg sodium, 6 g dietary fiber
Diet Exchanges: 4 ¹⁄₂ vegetable, 1 fat
Carb Choices: 2

OVEN-ROASTED BRUSSELS SPROUTS

Prep time: 10 minutes • Cook time: 18 minutes

1½   pounds Brussels sprouts, quartered

1   tablespoon olive oil

½   teaspoon salt

⅛   teaspoon freshly ground black pepper

4   cloves garlic, sliced

Preheat the oven to 400°F. Coat a baking sheet with cooking spray.

In a large bowl, combine the Brussels sprouts and oil. Spread in a single layer on the baking sheet. Sprinkle with salt and pepper. Roast the Brussels sprouts, shaking the pan occasionally, for 10 minutes. Remove the baking sheet from the oven and stir in the garlic. Return to the oven and roast for 8 to 10 minutes longer, or until the Brussels sprouts are tender and the edges are lightly browned.

Makes 4 servings

Per serving: 108 calories, 6 g protein, 16 g carbohydrates, 4 g fat, 0 mg cholesterol, 330 mg sodium, 7 g dietary fiber
Diet Exchanges: 3 vegetable, 1 fat
Carb Choices: 1

CAJUN-SPICED OVEN FRIES

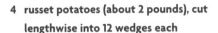

Prep time: 10 minutes • Cook time: 35 minutes

4 russet potatoes (about 2 pounds), cut lengthwise into 12 wedges each

1½ tablespoons olive oil

1 teaspoon chili powder

1 teaspoon ground cumin

1 teaspoon sweet paprika

1 teaspoon dried oregano

¼ teaspoon dried thyme

1 teaspoon salt

⅛ teaspoon cayenne pepper

Preheat the oven to 450°F. Coat a baking sheet with cooking spray.

In a large bowl, combine the potatoes and oil. Toss well to coat. In a small bowl, combine the chili powder, cumin, paprika, oregano, thyme, salt, and cayenne pepper. Sprinkle the spice mixture over the potatoes, tossing well to coat.

Arrange the potato wedges in a single layer on the baking sheet. Bake for 20 minutes. Turn the potatoes over and bake for 15 to 17 minutes longer, until crisp.

Makes 4 servings

Per serving: 109 calories, 5 g protein, 12 g carbohydrates, 5 g fat, 0 mg cholesterol, 610 mg sodium, 6 g dietary fiber
Diet Exchanges: 1 bread, 1 fat
Carb Choices: 1

QUINOA WITH RAISINS, APRICOTS, AND PECANS

Photo on page 126.

Prep time: 15 minutes • Cook time: 20 minutes

3 **tablespoons pecans, chopped**

⅔ **cup quinoa**

⅔ **cup orange juice**

⅔ **cup water**

⅓ **cup chopped dried apricots**

¼ **cup golden raisins**

2 **scallions, finely chopped**

1 **tablespoon chopped fresh cilantro**

1 **tablespoon lemon juice**

1 **tablespoon olive oil**

½ **teaspoon salt**

Cook the pecans in a small nonstick skillet over medium heat, stirring often, for 3 to 4 minutes, or until lightly toasted. Tip onto a plate and let cool.

Place the quinoa in a fine-mesh strainer and rinse under cold running water for 2 minutes. In a medium saucepan, combine the quinoa, orange juice, and water. Bring to a boil over high heat, reduce the heat to medium-low, cover, and simmer for 12 to 15 minutes, or until the liquid is absorbed. Transfer the quinoa to a large bowl. Add the apricots, raisins, scallions, cilantro, and toasted pecans. Add the lemon juice, oil, and salt, tossing well to distribute.

Makes 4 servings

Per serving: 266 calories, 5 g protein, 42 g carbohydrates, 9 g fat, 0 mg cholesterol, 300 mg sodium, 4 g dietary fiber
Diet Exchanges: 1 ½ fruit, 1 ½ bread, 1 ½ fat
Carb Choices: 3

BROWN BASMATI FRIED RICE

Prep time: 25 minutes • Cook time: 57 minutes • Stand time: 15 minutes

⅔ cup brown basmati rice	2 scallions, cut into ¼" pieces
2 tablespoons sesame oil	¼ pound snow peas, trimmed
1 egg, lightly beaten	½ cup frozen peas and carrots, thawed
2 teaspoons grated fresh ginger	3 tablespoons reduced-sodium soy sauce
1 teaspoon minced garlic	

In a medium saucepan, cook the rice according to package directions. Fluff the rice with a fork, spread it onto a baking sheet, and allow to cool for at least 15 minutes.

Heat 1 tablespoon of the oil in a large nonstick skillet over medium-high heat. Add the egg and cook, stirring, for 2 minutes, or until firm. Transfer to a bowl and reserve. Heat the remaining 1 tablespoon oil and add the ginger, garlic, scallions, and snow peas to the skillet. Cook, stirring often, for 2 minutes. Add the peas and carrots and the rice and cook for 2 to 3 minutes, or until the vegetables are crisp-tender. Add the soy sauce and cook for 3 to 5 minutes longer, or until the rice is heated through.

Makes 4 servings

Per serving: 228 calories, 6 g protein, 32 g carbohydrates, 9 g fat, 45 mg cholesterol, 530 mg sodium, 4 g dietary fiber
Diet Exchanges: ½ vegetable, 1½ bread, 1½ fat
Carb Choices: 2

TANGY LENTILS VINAIGRETTE

Prep time: 15 minutes • **Cook time: 18 minutes**

½ medium onion, root end trimmed but intact

3 cloves garlic

1 bay leaf

4 cups water

1 cup brown lentils, picked over

½ cup finely chopped red onion

½ cup chopped carrots

½ cup chopped celery

½ cup chopped red bell pepper

¼ cup chopped fresh basil

1 tablespoon capers, drained

3 tablespoons balsamic vinegar

2 tablespoons olive oil

½ teaspoon salt

¼ teaspoon freshly ground black pepper

In a large saucepan, combine the onion, garlic, and bay leaf with the water. Bring the water to a boil over medium-high heat. Add the lentils, reduce the heat to medium, and simmer for 18 to 20 minutes, or until tender. Drain the lentils and discard the onion, garlic, and bay leaf.

Transfer the lentils to a large bowl and stir in the red onion, carrots, celery, bell pepper, basil, and capers, tossing well to combine. Add the vinegar, oil, salt, and pepper. Mix well and serve at room temperature or chill to serve cold later.

Makes 4 servings

Per serving: 266 calories, 15 g protein, 37 g carbohydrates, 8 g fat, 0 mg cholesterol, 390 mg sodium, 17 g dietary fiber
Diet Exchanges: 1 vegetable, 2 bread, ½ meat, 1 ½ fat
Carb Choices: 2

MEDITERRANEAN COUSCOUS

Prep time: 15 minutes • Cook time: 7 minutes • Stand time: 10 minutes

1 ¼ cups water

¾ cup whole wheat couscous

½ teaspoon salt

½ cup canned red kidney beans, rinsed and drained

½ medium cucumber, peeled, seeded, and chopped

½ green bell pepper, chopped

¼ red onion, chopped

½ cup reduced-fat feta cheese

2 tablespoons chopped fresh dill

1 tablespoon capers, drained

2 tablespoons lemon juice

1 tablespoon olive oil

¼ teaspoon freshly ground black pepper

Bring the water to a boil in a medium saucepan over medium-high heat. Stir in the couscous and ¼ teaspoon of the salt. Return to a boil, reduce the heat to low, cover, and simmer for 2 minutes. Remove from the heat and let stand for 5 minutes. Fluff with a fork and cool for 5 minutes longer.

Meanwhile, in a bowl, combine the kidney beans, cucumber, bell pepper, onion, feta, dill, and capers. Add the couscous and toss well. In a small bowl, combine the lemon juice, olive oil, pepper, and the remaining ¼ teaspoon salt. Pour over the couscous and toss well.

Note: This recipe can be made up to 1 day ahead. Store it in an airtight plastic container in your refrigerator.

Makes 4 servings

Per serving: 244 calories, 11 g protein, 41 g carbohydrates, 6 g fat, 5 mg cholesterol, 590 mg sodium, 7 g dietary fiber
Diet Exchanges: ½ vegetable, 2 ½ bread, 1 meat, 1 fat
Carb Choices: 3

ROMAN PASTA CON PECORINO

Prep time: 5 minutes • Cook time: 15 minutes

8 ounces whole wheat spaghetti

7 tablespoons grated pecorino Romano cheese

2 tablespoons chopped fresh parsley

1 tablespoon olive oil

$\frac{1}{4}$ teaspoon crushed red-pepper flakes

$\frac{1}{4}$ teaspoon salt

$\frac{1}{8}$ teaspoon freshly ground black pepper

Bring a large pot of lightly salted water to a boil. Add the pasta and cook according to package directions. Drain the pasta, reserving $\frac{1}{2}$ cup of the cooking water. Transfer pasta to a large bowl. Add 6 tablespoons of the cheese, the parsley, oil, pepper flakes, salt, and pepper. Toss well, adding the pasta water, 1 tablespoon at a time, until the desired consistency is reached. Divide among 4 serving bowls. Sprinkle the dishes with the remaining 1 tablespoon cheese.

Makes 4 servings

Per serving: 272 calories, 12 g protein, 43 g carbohydrates, 7 g fat, 10 mg cholesterol, 280 mg sodium, 7 g dietary fiber
Diet Exchanges: $2\frac{1}{2}$ bread, $\frac{1}{2}$ meat, 1 fat
Carb Choices: 3

SOBA NOODLES WITH PEANUT SAUCE

Prep time: 10 minutes • Cook time: 15 minutes

3 **tablespoons peanut butter**

2 **tablespoons water**

1 **tablespoon honey**

1 **tablespoon rice vinegar**

1 **tablespoon reduced-sodium soy sauce**

1 **teaspoon grated fresh ginger**

1 **teaspoon sesame oil**

$\frac{1}{8}$ **teaspoon crushed red-pepper flakes**

4 **ounces soba or whole wheat noodles**

2 **carrots, cut into small matchsticks**

2 **scallions, chopped**

In a small saucepan over medium-high heat, combine the peanut butter, water, honey, vinegar, soy sauce, ginger, oil, and pepper flakes. Bring to a boil and cook, stirring constantly, for 1 minute. Set aside and keep warm.

Bring a pot of water to a boil. Add the noodles and return to a boil. Cook the noodles for 4 minutes, then stir in the carrots. Cook for 2 minutes longer, or until the carrots are crisp-tender. Drain the noodles and transfer to a large bowl. Toss with the scallions and peanut sauce. Serve immediately.

Makes 4 servings

Per serving: 195 calories, 7 g protein, 33 g carbohydrates, 5 g fat, 0 mg cholesterol, 420 mg sodium, 2 g dietary fiber
Diet Exchanges: 1 vegetable, 1 $\frac{1}{2}$ bread, $\frac{1}{2}$ meat, 1 fat
Carb Choices: 2

SATISFYING BEEF AND PORK MAIN DISHES

FAST ■ SUPER FAST ■ FAST PREP

GRILLED PEPPERED STEAK WITH MULTIGRAIN TEXAS TOAST

Prep time: 10 minutes • Cook time: 14 minutes

2 slices multigrain bread

½ teaspoon olive oil

1 clove garlic

½ pound lean boneless sirloin steak, trimmed of all visible fat

¾ teaspoon cracked tricolor peppercorns

2 tablespoons barbecue sauce

2 tablespoons prepared white horseradish sauce

½ tomato, cut into 4 slices

Preheat the oven to 425°F.

Brush 1 side of each slice of bread with the oil. Place oiled side up on a baking sheet and bake for 7 to 8 minutes, or until golden and crisp. Remove from the oven and rub the oiled side lightly with the garlic. Discard the leftover garlic and keep the toast warm.

Place the steak on a plate or work surface and press the peppercorns onto both sides. Coat a grill pan with cooking spray and heat over medium heat. Grill the steak for 3 minutes, then turn and brush with 1 tablespoon of the barbecue sauce. Grill for 3 minutes longer, then turn the steak over and brush with the remaining barbecue sauce. Grill 1 minute longer, or until an instant-read thermometer inserted into the center registers 145°F for medium-rare.

Remove from the grill and slice the steak. Spread 1 tablespoon horseradish sauce on each toasted bread slice and top with half of the sliced steak. Top each steak with 2 tomato slices.

Makes 2 servings

Per serving: 330 calories, 28 g protein, 19 g carbohydrates, 5 g fat, 80 mg cholesterol, 420 mg sodium, 2 g dietary fiber
Diet Exchanges: ½ vegetable, 1 bread, 2 ½ meat, ½ fat
Carb Choices: 1

BEEF TENDERLOIN STEAKS WITH MUSTARD-HORSERADISH SAUCE

Prep time: 7 minutes • Cook time: 7 minutes

SAUCE

3 tablespoons reduced-fat sour cream

1 small plum tomato, finely chopped

2 tablespoons snipped fresh chives or scallion greens

1 tablespoon prepared white horseradish

1 small shallot, minced

1 teaspoon grainy mustard

STEAKS

4 boneless beef tenderloin steaks (4 ounces each), well-trimmed

$^3/_4$ teaspoon coarsely ground black pepper

$^1/_4$ teaspoon salt

1 tablespoon grainy mustard

To make the sauce: In a small bowl, mix the sour cream, plum tomato, chives or scallion greens, horseradish, shallot, and mustard until well blended.

To make the steaks: Preheat the broiler. Coat a broiler-pan rack with olive oil cooking spray.

Sprinkle the steaks on both sides with the pepper and salt. Place on the prepared broiler pan. Broil 2" to 4" from the heat for 4 to 5 minutes, until browned. Turn and spread the tops with the mustard. Cook 3 to 4 minutes longer for medium-rare, or until done the way you like them.

Remove from the heat, transfer to a plate, and let stand for 5 minutes. Serve the steaks with the sauce.

Makes 4 servings

Per serving: 200 calories, 26 g protein, 3 g carbohydrates, 9 g fat, 80 mg cholesterol, 290 mg sodium, 0 g dietary fiber
Diet Exchanges: 3 $^1/_2$ meat, 1 $^1/_2$ fat
Carb Choices: 0

CHINO-LATINO BEEF KEBABS

Photo on page 127.

Prep time: 20 minutes • **Marinating time: 2 hours** • **Cook time: 8 minutes**

1 pound lean boneless sirloin, trimmed of all visible fat

1 tablespoon grated fresh ginger

2 cloves garlic, minced

3 tablespoons reduced-sodium soy sauce

1 teaspoon Worcestershire sauce

1 teaspoon dried oregano

½ teaspoon ground cumin

½ teaspoon sesame oil

1 sweet onion, such as Vidalia, cut into 16 pieces

1 medium green bell pepper, seeded and cut into 16 squares

12 cherry tomatoes

¼ teaspoon salt

With a sharp knife, cut the sirloin into twenty 1" cubes and place in a bowl. In a separate bowl, combine the ginger, garlic, soy sauce, Worcestershire sauce, oregano, cumin, and oil. Add the mixture to the beef and stir well to coat. Cover the bowl and refrigerate for 2 hours or overnight.

Preheat the broiler and coat a broiler-pan rack with cooking spray. Alternately thread 5 beef cubes, 4 onion pieces, 4 bell pepper squares, and 3 cherry tomatoes onto each of four 18" wooden or metal skewers. Place the skewers onto the broiler pan and sprinkle with the salt. Broil 4" from the heat source for 8 to 10 minutes, turning them every 2 minutes, until the vegetables are tender and the beef is cooked through.

Makes 4 servings

Per serving: 188 calories, 23 g protein, 9 g carbohydrates, 7 g fat, 65 mg cholesterol, 360 mg sodium, 2 g dietary fiber
Diet Exchanges: 2 vegetable, 3 meat, 1 fat
Carb Choices: 1

BEEF FAJITAS

Prep time: 15 minutes • Marinating time: 4 hours • Cook time: 18 minutes

1 tablespoon olive oil

4 cloves garlic, minced

2 tablespoons lime juice

1 teaspoon grated lime zest

1 teaspoon ground cumin

1 pound lean round tip sirloin, trimmed of all visible fat

¼ teaspoon salt

2 bell peppers, green or red, seeded and cut into ¼"-wide strips

1 onion, cut into ¼"-wide slices

4 whole wheat tortillas (8" diameter)

½ cup medium-hot salsa

¼ cup fat-free sour cream

In a resealable plastic bag, combine the oil, garlic, lime juice, lime zest, and cumin. Add the sirloin and toss well to coat. Refrigerate for 4 hours or overnight.

Preheat the grill or broiler. Remove the sirloin from the marinade, reserving any leftover marinade, and sprinkle with the salt. Grill or broil 4" from the heat for 5 to 6 minutes per side, or until an instant-read thermometer inserted into the center registers 145°F for medium-rare. Transfer to a cutting board and cover loosely with foil.

Heat a nonstick skillet over medium-high heat. Add the bell peppers, onion, and the reserved marinade. Cook, stirring often, for 8 to 9 minutes, or until the vegetables are softened. Warm the tortillas according to package directions.

Thinly slice the sirloin across the grain on a slight angle. To assemble a fajita, place 1 tortilla on a plate and top with one-quarter of the sirloin, one-quarter of the vegetable mixture, 2 tablespoons salsa, and 1 tablespoon sour cream. Repeat with the remaining ingredients.

Makes 4 servings

Per serving: 330 calories, 30 g protein, 33 g carbohydrates, 11 g fat, 50 mg cholesterol, 620 mg sodium, 4 g dietary fiber
Diet Exchanges: 2 vegetable, 1 bread, 3 ½ meat, 1 ½ fat
Carb Choices: 2

SUPER-EASY BARBECUE PULLED PORK

Prep time: 10 minutes • Cook time: 1 hour 45 minutes

1 tablespoon olive oil

1 ½ pounds boneless pork loin, trimmed of all visible fat

1 medium onion, chopped (about ½ cup)

⅔ cup ketchup

1 tablespoon cider vinegar

1 tablespoon molasses

2 teaspoons packed brown sugar

2 teaspoons mustard powder

1 ½ teaspoons garlic powder

1 teaspoon Worcestershire sauce

¼ teaspoon freshly ground black pepper

1 ½ cups chicken or vegetable broth

Heat the oil in a medium saucepan over medium-high heat. Add the pork loin and brown, turning occasionally, for 5 minutes. Add the onion, ketchup, vinegar, molasses, sugar, mustard powder, garlic powder, Worcestershire sauce, black pepper, and broth. Stir the mixture well to combine and bring to a boil over medium-high heat. Reduce the heat to low, cover, and simmer, stirring occasionally, for 1 ½ hours. Uncover the saucepan and simmer 10 minutes longer, or until the sauce has thickened slightly and the pork is very tender. Remove from the heat.

Pull the pork into shreds with two forks and serve.

Makes 6 servings

Per serving: 249 calories, 26 g protein, 18 g carbohydrates, 8 g fat, 75 mg cholesterol, 630 mg sodium, 1 g dietary fiber
Diet Exchanges: ½ vegetable, 1 bread, 3 ½ meat, 1 fat
Carb Choices: 1

GRILLED PORK TENDERLOIN WITH GRILLED PEACHES

Prep time: 8 minutes • Cook time: 26 minutes

1 whole pork tenderloin (1 pound), trimmed	½ teaspoon freshly ground black pepper
1½ teaspoons sweet paprika	¼ teaspoon cayenne pepper
½ teaspoon mustard powder	2 tablespoons canola oil
½ teaspoon salt	2 large firm-ripe peaches or nectarines

Heat a barbecue grill to medium.

Place the pork tenderloin on a rimmed baking sheet. In a cup, mix the paprika, mustard powder, salt, and peppers. Rub all over the pork. Spoon 1 tablespoon of the oil over the pork and roll it gently in the pan so all sides are coated.

Place the pork on the grill rack. Cover and grill, turning once or twice, for 20 to 25 minutes, or until an instant-read thermometer inserted into the thickest part registers 155°F. Transfer to a platter and cover loosely to keep warm.

Meanwhile, halve and pit the peaches, and brush the insides and outsides with the remaining 1 tablespoon oil.

Place the peach halves on the grill cut side up. Grill, moving them a few times, for 6 to 10 minutes, depending on the ripeness, until the color deepens and the fruit feels soft.

Cut the pork into thin slices and serve with the grilled peaches.

Makes 4 servings

Per serving: 230 calories, 25 g protein, 8 g carbohydrates, 11 g fat, 75 mg cholesterol, 350 mg sodium, 1 g dietary fiber
Diet Exchanges: ½ fruit, 3½ meat, 2 fat
Carb Choices: ½

ROASTED PORK LOIN WITH ORANGE AND THYME

Prep time: 6 minutes • Cook time: 50 minutes

3 cloves garlic

2 teaspoons grated orange zest

¾ teaspoon dried thyme

½ teaspoon salt

½ teaspoon freshly ground black pepper

¼ teaspoon crushed red-pepper flakes

1 center-cut boneless pork-loin roast (1 pound), well-trimmed

Orange wedges or slices

Preheat the oven to 375°F. Line a 9" × 9" baking pan with foil and coat the foil with olive oil cooking spray.

On a cutting board, combine the garlic, orange zest, thyme, salt, black pepper, and red-pepper flakes. Chop together until the garlic is finely minced and the ingredients are well blended. Rub all over the pork.

Place the pork in the prepared pan. Roast for 50 to 60 minutes, or until an instant-read thermometer inserted in the thickest part registers 155°F.

Remove the pork from the oven and let it stand for 10 minutes before carving into thin slices. Serve with orange wedges or slices as a garnish.

Makes 4 servings

Per serving: 170 calories, 25 g protein, 1 g carbohydrates, 7 g fat, 70 mg cholesterol, 370 mg sodium, 0 g dietary fiber
Diet Exchanges: 3 ½ meat, 1 fat
Carb Choices: 0

LOIN PORK CHOPS BRAISED WITH PORT AND PRUNES

Prep time: 10 minutes • Cook time: 23 minutes

16 pitted prunes, chopped	**¼ cup finely chopped celery**
¾ cup port wine	**1 teaspoon chopped fresh thyme**
4 boneless loin pork chops (4 ounces each)	**½ cup reduced-sodium, fat-free beef broth**
½ teaspoon salt	**1 tablespoon red currant jelly or apricot preserves**
1 tablespoon butter	
¼ cup finely chopped leeks	**⅛ teaspoon freshly ground black pepper**
¼ cup finely chopped carrots	

In a medium saucepan, combine the prunes and port. Bring to a simmer over medium-low heat and simmer for 7 to 10 minutes, or until the prunes are plump, then remove from the heat.

Sprinkle the pork chops with ¼ teaspoon of the salt. In a large nonstick skillet over medium-high heat, melt ½ tablespoon of the butter and add the pork chops. Cook for 1 minute per side, or until lightly browned. Remove the pork from the pan.

Reduce the heat to medium and add the leeks, carrots, celery, and thyme to the skillet. Cook, stirring occasionally, for 4 to 5 minutes, or until the vegetables are lightly browned. Add the beef broth and the prune mixture to the skillet and bring to a simmer over medium-low heat. Place the pork in the skillet and cook for 4 to 5 minutes, or until the pork is tender and cooked through. Remove the pork chops to a plate and keep warm.

Increase the heat under the skillet to high and bring to a boil. Boil the sauce for 3 to 4 minutes, or until it starts to thicken slightly. Remove from the heat and stir in the jelly or preserves, pepper, and the remaining ½ tablespoon butter and ¼ teaspoon salt. Spoon the sauce and prunes over the pork and serve.

Makes 4 servings

Per serving: 400 calories, 27 g protein, 37 g carbohydrates, 10 g fat, 70 mg cholesterol, 390 mg sodium, 2 g dietary fiber
Diet Exchanges: 2 fruit, ½ vegetable, 3 ½ meat, 2 ½ fat
Carb Choices: 2

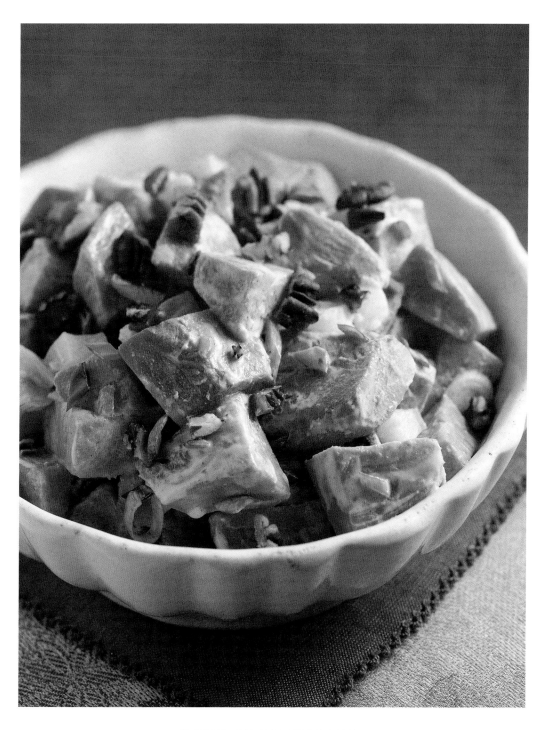

CURRIED SWEET POTATO SALAD

Recipe on page 74

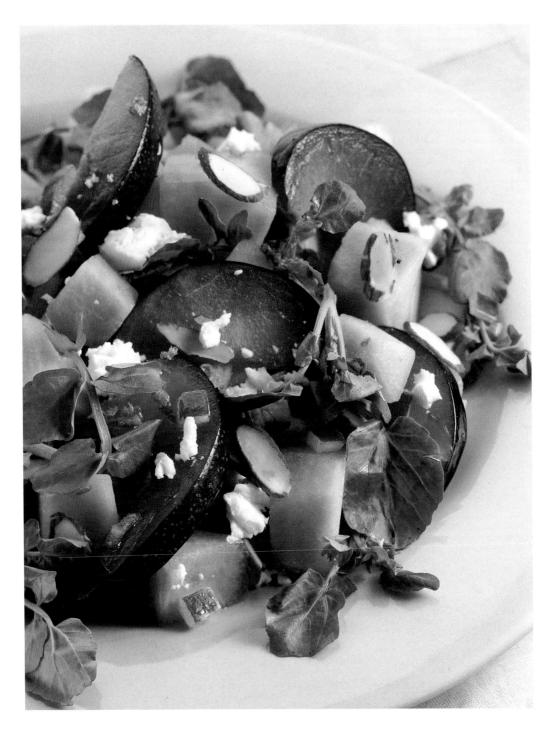

CANTALOUPE AND WATERCRESS SALAD WITH PICKLED ONIONS

Recipe on page 76

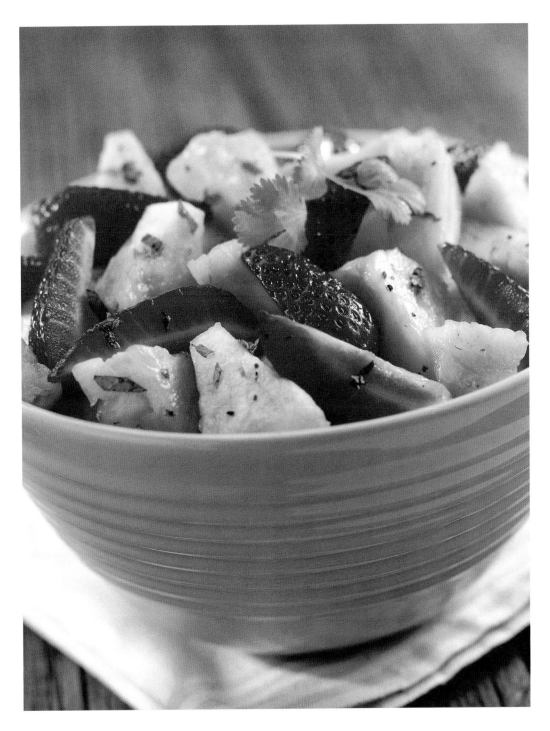

PINEAPPLE AND STRAWBERRIES WITH CILANTRO AND PEPPER

Recipe on page 78

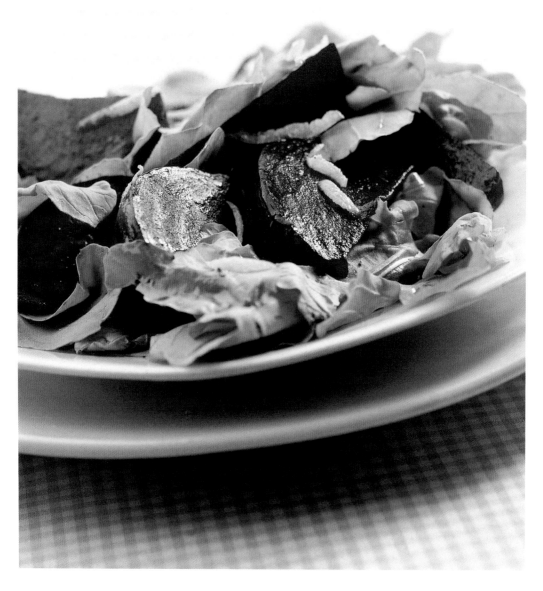

ANISE-SCENTED BALSAMIC BEETS

Recipe on page 98

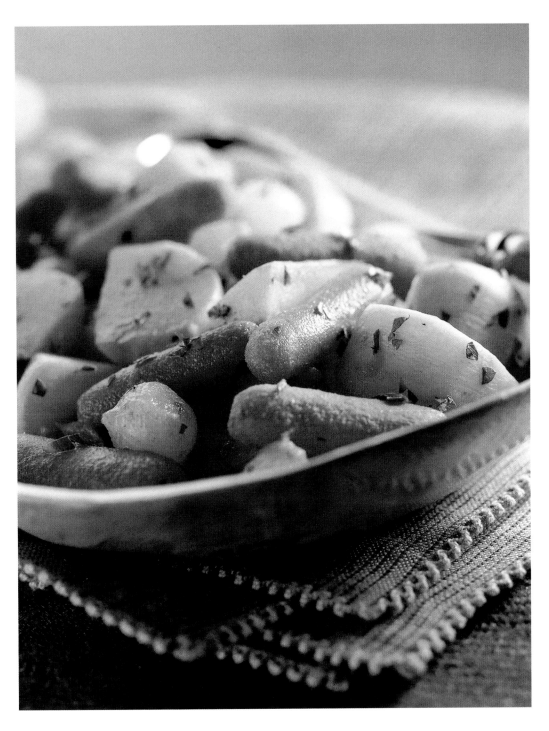

GLAZED TURNIPS, PEARL ONIONS, AND CARROTS

Recipe on page 103

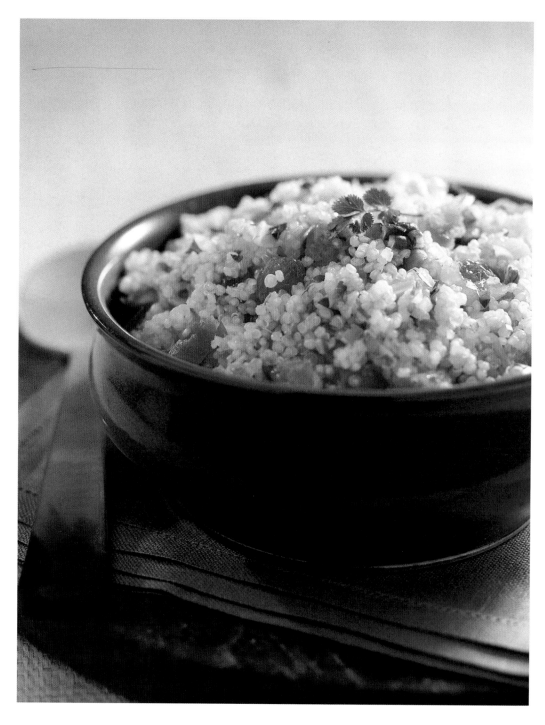

QUINOA WITH RAISINS, APRICOTS, AND PECANS

Recipe on page 106

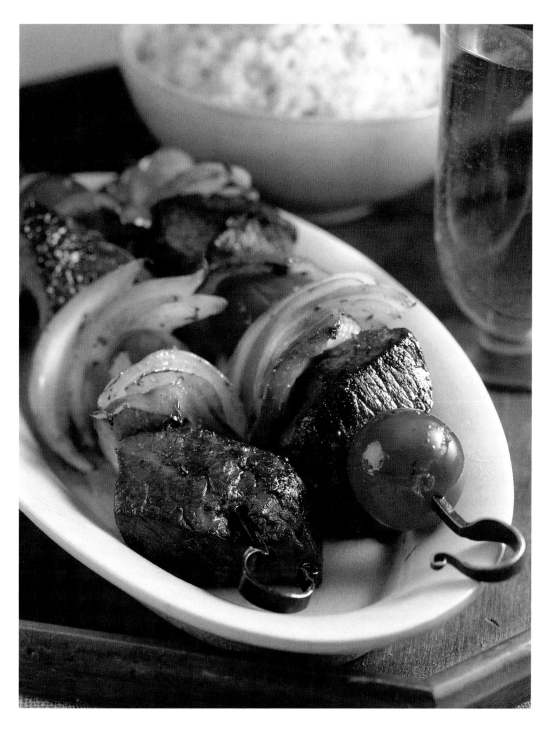

CHINO-LATINO BEEF KEBABS

Recipe on page 115

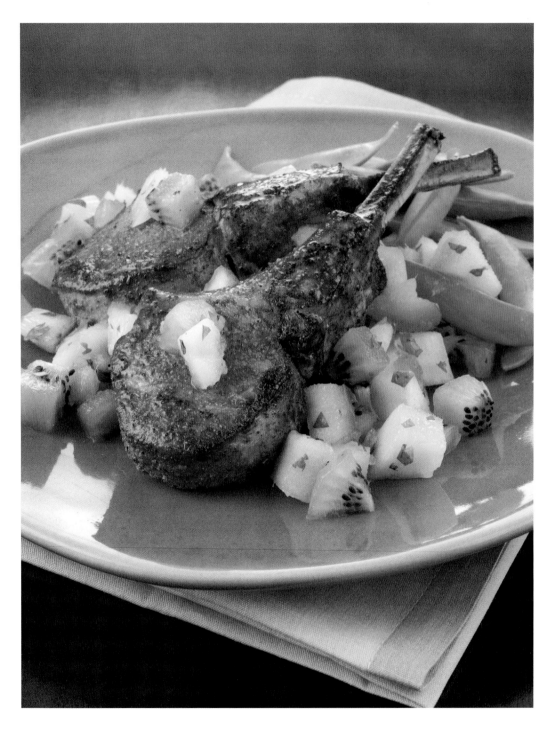

SPICED LAMB CHOPS WITH MANGO-KIWI RELISH

Recipe on page 129

SPICED LAMB CHOPS WITH MANGO-KIWI RELISH

Photo on page 128.

FAST

Prep time: 12 minutes • Cook time: 10 minutes

4 bone-in rib or loin lamb chops (5 to 6 ounces each), well trimmed

$\frac{1}{2}$ teaspoon ground cumin

$\frac{1}{2}$ teaspoon ground ginger

$\frac{1}{4}$ teaspoon turmeric

$\frac{1}{8}$ teaspoon ground nutmeg

$\frac{1}{8}$ teaspoon ground cinnamon

$\frac{1}{2}$ teaspoon salt

$\frac{1}{2}$ teaspoon freshly ground black pepper

$\frac{1}{4}$ teaspoon sugar

1 ripe mango, peeled and chopped

2 ripe kiwifruits, peeled and chopped

2 tablespoons chopped fresh mint leaves

If the chops are thick, pound them a little with the flat side of a chef's knife or the flat side of a meat mallet, so that they cook more evenly.

In a cup, mix the cumin, ginger, turmeric, nutmeg, cinnamon, salt, pepper, and sugar. Rub the spice mixture over both sides of the chops. Put the chops on a plate, cover loosely, and let stand while making the mango relish. (This can be done earlier in the day, and the chops refrigerated.)

Preheat the broiler.

In a small bowl, mix the mango, kiwifruits, and mint. Cover and set aside.

Broil the lamb chops 4" from the heat for 5 to 6 minutes per side, turning once, for medium. Serve the chops with the mango-kiwi relish.

Makes 4 servings

Per serving: 250 calories, 31 g protein, 15 g carbohydrates, 7 g fat, 115 mg cholesterol, 360 mg sodium, 3 g dietary fiber
Diet Exchanges: 1 fruit, 4 $\frac{1}{2}$ meat
Carb Choices: 1

HERBED BUTTERFLIED LEG OF LAMB

Prep time: 10 minutes • Marinating time: 2 to 3 hours, or overnight • Cook time: 30 minutes

¼ cup dry red wine

1 tablespoon extra-virgin olive oil

2 tablespoons coarsely chopped fresh rosemary

2 bay leaves

¾ teaspoon dried oregano, crumbled

¾ teaspoon dried mint, crumbled

½ teaspoon coarse-ground black pepper

1 butterflied leg of lamb (2 pounds), well-trimmed

¾ teaspoon salt

In a shallow glass dish, stir together the wine, oil, rosemary, bay leaves, oregano, mint, and pepper. Add the lamb and turn to coat with the marinade. Cover and marinate in the refrigerator for 2 to 3 hours or overnight, turning once or twice.

Preheat a barbecue grill to medium. Remove the lamb from the dish, reserving the marinade, and sprinkle both sides with the salt. Place the lamb on the grill rack and spoon some of the reserved marinade over. Discard the remaining marinade and bay leaves.

Cover the lamb and grill, turning 2 or 3 times, and moving it away from any hot spots, for 20 to 30 minutes, or until an instant-read thermometer inserted into the thickest part registers 145°F for medium-rare (the edges will be crispy and more well done).

Place the lamb on a platter to catch the juices and let stand for 10 minutes. Cut into thin slices.

Makes 8 servings

Per serving: 310 calories, 20 g protein, 0 g carbohydrates, 24 g fat, 75 mg cholesterol, 300 mg sodium, 0 g dietary fiber
Diet Exchanges: 3 meat, 3 ½ fat
Carb Choices: 0

HEALTHY POULTRY AND SEAFOOD MAIN DISHES

■ FAST   ■ SUPER FAST   ■ FAST PREP

GRILLED CHICKEN AND BROCCOLI RABE
WITH GARLIC-PARSLEY SAUCE

Prep time: 15 minutes • Cook time: 12 minutes

SAUCE

1 cup loosely packed flat-leaf parsley sprigs

3 tablespoons lemon juice

2 tablespoons extra-virgin olive oil

2 tablespoons reduced-sodium chicken or
   vegetable broth, or water

1 tablespoon fresh oregano leaves

1 clove garlic

¼ teaspoon salt

⅛ teaspoon cayenne pepper (optional)

¼ cup finely chopped red bell pepper

CHICKEN AND BROCCOLI RABE

4 boneless, skinless chicken breast halves,
   trimmed

1 package (12 ounces) microwaveable cut
   broccoli rabe

To make the sauce: In a food processor or blender, combine the parsley, lemon juice, oil, broth or water, oregano, garlic, salt, and cayenne pepper, if using. Process until nearly smooth, stopping the machine once or twice to scrape down the sides. Transfer to a small bowl and stir in the bell pepper.

To make the chicken and broccoli rabe: Place the chicken in a pie plate and spoon 3 tablespoons of the garlic-parsley sauce over. Turn to coat, cover, and let stand while heating a barbecue grill to medium-hot.

Grill the chicken, covered, turning once, for 8 minutes, or until lightly charred and no longer pink in the thickest part. Transfer to a clean plate and cover loosely with foil to keep warm.

Microwave the broccoli rabe according to the package instructions. Divide among 4 plates, and place a chicken breast on top. Spoon the remaining sauce over and serve.

Makes 4 servings (½ cup sauce)

Per serving: 220 calories, 30 g protein, 6 g carbohydrates, 9 g fat, 65 mg cholesterol, 270 mg sodium, 2 g dietary fiber
Diet Exchanges: 1½ vegetable, 4 meat, 1½ fat
Carb Choices: ½

PEKING CHICKEN WRAPS

Photo on page 153.

Prep time: 30 minutes • **Cook time: 35 minutes**

½ cup brown rice

2 teaspoons dark sesame oil

4 scallions, sliced

¼ pound snow peas, trimmed

1 cup finely shredded red cabbage

1 cup shredded carrot

2 tablespoons unseasoned rice vinegar

2 teaspoons grated fresh ginger

6 whole wheat tortillas (10"–12" diameter)

6 tablespoons hoisin sauce

2 cups shredded cooked chicken breast

Cook the rice according to the package directions. Set aside.

Meanwhile, in a medium nonstick skillet, heat the oil over medium-high heat. Add the scallions and cook, stirring constantly, for 1 minute, or until wilted. Stir into the rice.

Bring a small pot of water to a boil. Add the snow peas and cook for 30 seconds. Drain and rinse with cold water until cool. Pat dry and cut lengthwise into thin strips. In a medium bowl, combine the snow peas, cabbage, carrot, rice vinegar, and ginger.

To assemble the wraps, lay the tortillas on a work surface. Spread each with 1 tablespoon hoisin sauce. Place one-sixth of the chicken in a strip along the bottom of each tortilla, 1" from the edges. Top with the rice and vegetable mixtures. Fold over the bottom edge of each tortilla to cover the filling. Fold the sides in and continue to roll up tightly, burrito style. Cut each in half crosswise with a serrated knife to serve.

Makes 6 servings

Per serving: 290 calories, 23 g protein, 45 g carbohydrates, 4 g fat, 45 mg cholesterol, 490 mg sodium, 5 g dietary fiber
Diet Exchanges: 1 vegetable, 2 ½ bread, 2 ½ meat, ½ fat
Carb Choices: 3

OVEN-"FRIED" CHICKEN

Prep time: 20 minutes • Chill time: 2 hours • Cook time: 50 minutes

1 **cut-up chicken (4 pounds), skin and any visible fat removed**

1 **cup buttermilk**

1 **clove garlic, minced**

2 **tablespoons ground flaxseed**

½ **cup dry whole wheat bread crumbs**

3 **tablespoons whole grain pastry flour**

3 **tablespoons cornmeal**

1 **teaspoon salt**

¾ **teaspoon freshly ground black pepper**

½ **teaspoon ground red pepper**

Cut the chicken breasts in half. In a large bowl, combine the buttermilk and garlic. Add the chicken and turn to coat. Cover and refrigerate for 2 hours or overnight.

Preheat the oven to 400°F. Coat a large jelly-roll pan with cooking spray.

In a large food storage bag, shake the ground flaxseed, bread crumbs, flour, cornmeal, salt, and black and red pepper until blended. Drain the chicken in a colander. Pick up the chicken one piece at a time, letting the excess buttermilk drip off. Add to the bag and shake to coat. Place the chicken skinned side up on the prepared pan. Coat the chicken with cooking spray.

Bake for 50 to 55 minutes, or until an instant-read thermometer inserted into the thickest portion registers 170°F and the juices run clear.

Makes 6 servings

Per serving: 258 calories, 35 g protein, 14 g carbohydrates, 6 g fat, 100 mg cholesterol, 560 mg sodium, 2 g dietary fiber
Diet Exchanges: 1 bread, 5 meat, ½ fat
Carb Choices: 1

CHICKEN PESTO PRESTO

Prep time: 5 minutes • Cook time: 6 minutes

3–4 plum tomatoes

½ cup shredded part-skim mozzarella
cheese

2 tablespoons grated Parmesan cheese

1 pound thinly sliced chicken breast
cutlets (8 pieces)

¼ teaspoon salt

¼ teaspoon crushed red-pepper flakes

2 tablespoons prepared pesto sauce

Preheat the broiler. Coat a rimmed baking sheet with olive oil cooking spray.

Thinly slice the tomatoes lengthwise, discarding the core and the outside slices, to get 16 slices. Mix the mozzarella and Parmesan in a small bowl.

Arrange the chicken cutlets on the prepared baking sheet. Sprinkle with the salt and red-pepper flakes, and spread each with equal amounts of pesto.

Broil the chicken 2" to 4" from the heat for 5 minutes, or until no longer pink in the thickest part and the edges are lightly browned.

Remove from the oven. Top each piece of chicken with 2 tomato slices, overlapping if necessary, and sprinkle evenly with the mixed cheeses. Broil for 1 to 2 minutes longer, just until the cheese is melted and the tomatoes are heated. Serve right away.

Makes 4 servings

Per serving: 210 calories, 29 g protein, 3 g carbohydrates, 8 g fat, 75 mg cholesterol, 730 mg sodium, 0 g dietary fiber
Diet Exchanges: 4 ½ meat, 1 fat, ½ vegetable
Carb Choices: 0

OSSO BUCO-STYLE CHICKEN

Prep time: 20 minutes • Cook time: 45 minutes

2 tablespoons olive oil

8 chicken drumsticks (2 pounds), skin removed

½ teaspoon salt

1 medium onion, chopped

2 carrots, chopped

2 ribs celery, chopped

4 cloves garlic, minced

1 can (14 ½ ounces) Italian-style diced tomatoes

1 can (14–19 ounces) chickpeas, rinsed and drained

1 cup chicken or vegetable broth

½ cup white wine or chicken broth

1 bay leaf

¼ cup chopped flat-leaf parsley

1 tablespoon grated lemon peel

In a soup pot or Dutch oven, heat the oil over medium-high heat. Sprinkle the chicken with ¼ teaspoon of the salt. Add the chicken and cook, turning occasionally, for 6 to 8 minutes, or until browned. Remove the chicken to a plate.

Reduce the heat to low and add the onion, carrots, celery, and the remaining ¼ teaspoon salt. Cover and cook for 8 minutes, or until the vegetables soften. Set aside 1 teaspoon garlic. Stir in the remaining garlic and cook for 1 minute. Add the tomatoes (with juice), chickpeas, broth, wine or broth, and bay leaf. Return the chicken to the pot. Bring to a boil. Reduce the heat, cover, and simmer for 30 to 35 minutes, or until the chicken is very tender. Remove and discard the bay leaf.

In a small bowl, combine the parsley, lemon peel, and the reserved 1 teaspoon garlic. Stir until combined. Serve the chicken sprinkled with the parsley mixture.

Makes 8 servings

Per serving: 276 calories, 28 g protein, 18 g carbohydrates, 9 g fat, 80 mg cholesterol, 670 mg sodium, 4 g dietary fiber
Diet Exchanges: 1 ½ vegetable, ½ bread, 3 ½ meat, 1 ½ fat
Carb Choices: 1

TANDOORI TURKEY CUTLETS
WITH PEAR-CHERRY CHUTNEY

Prep time: 15 minutes • Cook time: 4 minutes

1 **large ripe pear, peeled, cored, and chopped**

1 **cup pitted fresh or frozen and thawed cherries, quartered**

½ **small red bell pepper, chopped**

¼ **cup bottled mango chutney**

2 **tablespoons finely chopped red onion**

2 **tablespoons chopped cilantro (optional)**

1 **tablespoon lime juice**

1 **teaspoon curry powder**

1 **teaspoon paprika**

1 **teaspoon ground cumin**

¼ **teaspoon salt**

4 **turkey cutlets (4 ounces each)**

In a medium bowl, combine the pear, cherries, bell pepper, chutney, onion, cilantro (if using), and lime juice. Set aside.

In a small bowl, combine the curry powder, paprika, cumin, and salt. Sprinkle both sides of the turkey cutlets with the spice mixture, patting to coat.

Heat a grill pan over medium heat. Coat the pan with cooking spray. Cook the cutlets for 2 minutes on each side, or until no longer pink. Serve with the chutney.

Makes 4 servings (2 cups chutney)

Per serving: 223 calories, 27 g protein, 21 g carbohydrates, 4 g fat, 60 mg cholesterol, 200 mg sodium, 3 g dietary fiber
Diet Exchanges: 1 fruit, 1 vegetable, 4 meat
Carb Choices: 1

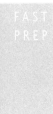

TURKEY AND BEAN CHILI

Prep time: 20 minutes • Cook time: 1 hour 10 minutes

1 **pound ground turkey breast**

1 **large onion, chopped**

2 **red or yellow bell peppers, chopped**

4 **large cloves garlic, minced**

3 **tablespoons tomato paste**

2 **tablespoons chili powder**

1 **tablespoon ground cumin**

1 **teaspoon dried oregano**

1 **teaspoon salt**

1 **large sweet potato, peeled and cut into $\frac{1}{2}$" cubes**

1 **can (28 ounces) diced tomatoes**

1 **can (14 ounces) chicken broth**

1 **chipotle chile pepper in adobo sauce, minced (optional)**

2 **cans (15–16 ounces each) mixed beans for chili, rinsed and drained**

1 **zucchini, chopped**

In a large soup pot or Dutch oven, over medium-high heat, cook the turkey, onion, and bell peppers, stirring frequently, for 8 minutes, or until the turkey is cooked through. Add the garlic, tomato paste, chili powder, cumin, oregano, and salt. Cook, stirring constantly, for 1 minute.

Add the sweet potato, diced tomatoes (with juice), chicken broth, and chipotle chile, if using. Bring to a boil. Reduce the heat to low and simmer, covered, stirring occasionally, for 30 minutes.

Stir in the beans and zucchini. Return to a simmer. Cover and simmer for 30 minutes longer, stirring occasionally, or until the flavors are well-blended and the vegetables are tender.

Makes 8 servings

Per serving: 227 calories, 17 g protein, 29 g carbohydrates, 5 g fat, 45 mg cholesterol, 680 mg sodium, 10 g dietary fiber
Diet Exchanges: 2 vegetable, 1 bread, 2 meat
Carb Choices: 2

SKILLET TURKEY TETRAZZINI

Photo on page 154.

Prep time: 20 minutes • Cook time: 30 minutes

½ pound whole wheat pasta, such as penne

1 bag (10 ounces) fresh spinach, large leaves torn in half

1 tablespoon olive oil

1 pound turkey cutlets, cut into ¾" pieces

1 box (8 ounces) sliced mushrooms

1 small onion, finely chopped

¾ cup chicken broth

¾ cup 1% milk

2 tablespoons cornstarch

½ cup frozen peas

¾ cup freshly grated Parmesan cheese

2 tablespoons ground flaxseed

Prepare the pasta according to package directions. Before draining, add the spinach and stir until wilted. Drain the pasta.

In a large ovenproof skillet, heat the oil over medium-high heat. Add the turkey and cook, stirring frequently, for 3 to 4 minutes, or until no longer pink. Remove to a plate.

Reduce the heat to medium-low and add the mushrooms and onion to the skillet. Cook, stirring frequently, for 5 minutes, or until softened. Add the chicken broth and bring to a boil.

Preheat the broiler. In a small bowl, combine the milk and cornstarch. Stir until the cornstarch dissolves. Stir into the broth mixture. Add the peas and bring to a boil, stirring frequently. Reduce the heat and simmer for 3 minutes, stirring frequently. Stir ½ cup of the cheese, turkey, and pasta into the sauce. Sprinkle with the flaxseed and remaining ¼ cup cheese. Broil for 2 to 3 minutes, or until the cheese melts.

Makes 6 servings

Per serving: 383 calories, 28 g protein, 39 g carbohydrates, 14 g fat, 70 mg cholesterol, 480 mg sodium, 8 g dietary fiber
Diet Exchanges: 1 vegetable, 2 bread, 3 ½ meat, 1 fat
Carb Choices: 3

BAKED ZITI WITH TURKEY SAUSAGE

Prep time: 15 minutes • Cook time: 50 minutes

1 ½ cups (5 ounces) whole wheat ziti, rotelle, or other short pasta

1 teaspoon + 2 tablespoons olive oil

1 pound lean Italian-style turkey sausage (mild or hot), cut into 4" pieces

1 large red bell pepper, chopped

1 small onion, chopped

6 large mushrooms (6 ounces), coarsely chopped

3 cloves garlic, minced

1 teaspoon dried oregano

½ teaspoon dried thyme

1 can (15 ounces) crushed tomatoes

¼ teaspoon salt

¼ teaspoon ground black pepper

1 large ripe tomato, chopped or cut into thin pieces (optional)

¾ cup (3 ounces) shredded mozzarella cheese

Preheat the oven to 375° F. Spray a shallow 3-quart baking dish with cooking spray and set aside.

Cook the pasta according to package directions. Drain and return to the pot. Add 1 teaspoon of the oil and toss to coat.

Heat the remaining 2 tablespoons oil in a large skillet over medium heat. Add the sausage and cook until browned and no longer pink inside, 8 to 10 minutes. Transfer the sausage to a clean plate and allow to cool while preparing the rest of the sauce.

Into the same skillet, add the bell pepper, onion, mushrooms, garlic, oregano, and thyme. Cook until the onion is almost soft, 6 to 7 minutes, stirring occasionally. Stir in the crushed tomatoes and cook for 5 minutes. Season with salt and black pepper.

Cut the sausage into ¼" slices and place in the prepared baking dish along with the sauce and pasta. Toss to combine. Top with fresh tomato (if using), only around the edges if desired, and sprinkle with the cheese. Bake until heated through and the cheese is melted and slightly browned, 20 to 25 minutes.

Makes 4 servings

Per serving: 340 calories, 26 g protein, 27 g carbohydrates, 15 g fat, 60 mg cholesterol, 293 mg sodium, 5 g fiber
Diet Exchanges: 2 vegetable, 1 bread, 3 meat, 2 ½ fat
Carb Choices: 2

STOVETOP-SMOKED TROUT WITH APPLE-HORSERADISH SAUCE

Prep time: 45 minutes • Chill time: 2 hours • Cook time: 25 minutes

SAUCE

¼ cup light mayonnaise

3 tablespoons reduced-fat sour cream

4 teaspoons prepared horseradish, drained

½ small Granny Smith apple, peeled and finely chopped

½ teaspoon Dijon mustard

TROUT

1 quart water

½ teaspoon salt

2 cloves garlic, minced

2 tablespoons packed brown sugar

2 tablespoons honey

4 trout fillets (4–6 ounces each)

1 cup mesquite wood chips, soaked in water for 30 minutes (see note)

¾ cup granulated sugar

¾ cup uncooked rice

To make the sauce: Combine the mayonnaise, sour cream, horseradish, apple, and mustard in a bowl. Refrigerate until ready to use.

To make the trout: In a large bowl, combine the water, salt, garlic, brown sugar, and honey. Add the trout and refrigerate for 2 hours.

In a small bowl, combine the wood chips, granulated sugar, and rice. Line a heavy Dutch oven or large cast-iron skillet with a double layer of heavy-duty aluminum foil. Spread the sugar mixture evenly over the bottom of the Dutch oven. Set a wire rack 1½" to 2" above the sugar mixture in the Dutch oven. Remove the trout from the salt solution and rinse with cold water.

Place the trout on the wire rack. Cover the Dutch oven and set over high heat. When the pan begins to smoke, reduce the heat to low and cook for 15 to 20 minutes. Remove from the heat and let stand for 4 minutes.

Note: Make sure you have a well-ventilated kitchen or a good exhaust fan before making this dish.

Makes 4 servings (¾ cup sauce)

Per serving: 280 calories, 24 g protein, 13 g carbohydrates, 14 g fat, 75 mg cholesterol, 510 mg sodium, 1 g dietary fiber
Diet Exchanges: 1 bread, 3 meat, 2 fat
Carb Choices: 1

ROSEMARY-SCENTED SWORDFISH KEBABS

Prep time: 10 minutes • Marinating time: 1 ½ hours • Cook time: 8 minutes

2 cloves garlic, minced

1 medium shallot, minced

2 tablespoons Dijon mustard

2 tablespoons orange juice

1 tablespoon chopped fresh rosemary

2 teaspoons olive oil

2 teaspoons grated orange zest

4 swordfish steaks (6 ounces each), about ¾" thick

½ teaspoon salt

¼ teaspoon freshly ground black pepper

In a medium bowl, combine the garlic, shallot, mustard, orange juice, rosemary, oil, and orange zest. Add the swordfish to the bowl and coat with the mustard mixture. Refrigerate for 1 ½ hours.

Preheat the grill to medium hot. Remove the swordfish from the marinade and wipe off the excess. Sprinkle the swordfish with the salt and pepper and grill for 4 to 5 minutes per side, or until the fish is cooked through.

Makes 4 servings

Per serving: 233 calories, 32 g protein, 3 g carbohydrates, 9 g fat, 60 mg cholesterol, 620 mg sodium, 0 g dietary fiber
Diet Exchanges: 4 ½ meat, 1 fat
Carb Choices: 0

DILLED SALMON EN PAPILLOTE

Prep time: 20 minutes • Cook time: 15 minutes

1 small onion, chopped

1 clove garlic, minced

1 package frozen spinach (10 ounces), thawed and excess liquid squeezed out

1 tablespoon + 2 teaspoons lemon juice

2 tablespoons chopped fresh dill

4 teaspoons Dijon mustard

4 salmon fillets (4 ounces each), skin and pinbones removed

$\frac{1}{2}$ teaspoon salt

$\frac{1}{8}$ teaspoon freshly ground black pepper

4 teaspoons drained capers

4 teaspoons light butter

Preheat the oven to 400°F. Coat 4 sheets of aluminum foil 12" × 20" with cooking spray. Fold the aluminum foil sheets in half crosswise.

Coat a medium skillet with cooking spray and heat over medium-high heat. Add the onion and garlic and cook for 1 minute. Add the spinach and cook for 2 minutes, or until hot. Add 1 tablespoon of the lemon juice and cook for 30 seconds, stirring. Remove from the heat and stir in 1 tablespoon of the dill. Cool for 10 minutes.

In a small bowl, combine the mustard and the remaining 1 tablespoon dill and 2 teaspoons lemon juice.

Sprinkle the salmon with the salt and the pepper. Unfold the foil sheets and place one-quarter of the spinach mixture on half of each sheet. Top each mound of spinach with 1 salmon fillet. Spread the mustard mixture over the tops and sides of each fillet. Sprinkle 1 teaspoon of the capers over each fillet. Top each fillet with 1 teaspoon of the butter. Fold the foil over the salmon and, starting at one end, crimp the edges of the foil together to make a tight seal.

Transfer the foil packets to a large baking sheet. Bake for 12 to 15 minutes, or until the packets are puffed (they may not all puff). Arrange on dinner plates and cut open at the table.

Makes 4 servings

Per serving: 207 calories, 19 g protein, 7 g carbohydrates, 12 g fat, 55 mg cholesterol, 650 mg sodium, 2 g dietary fiber
Diet Exchanges: 1 vegetable, 2 $\frac{1}{2}$ meat, 1 fat
Carb Choices: 1

TERIYAKI-GLAZED TUNA STEAKS WITH ASIAN SLAW

Prep time: 15 minutes • Cook time: 10 minutes

SLAW

½ small head napa cabbage	2 tablespoons rice vinegar
1 cup snow peas, trimmed	1 tablespoon reduced-sodium soy sauce
1 carrot, peeled and grated	2 teaspoons honey
1 scallion, chopped	¼ teaspoon sesame oil

TUNA STEAKS

2 teaspoons cornstarch	⅛ teaspoon crushed red-pepper flakes
¼ cup orange juice	2 teaspoons sesame oil
3 tablespoons reduced-sodium soy sauce	4 yellowfin tuna steaks (6 ounces each), about ¾" thick
5 teaspoons honey	

To make the slaw: Using a sharp knife, thinly shred the cabbage (yielding about 4 cups) and transfer to a large bowl. Cut the snow peas into thin strips and add to the cabbage along with the carrot and scallion. Add the vinegar, soy sauce, honey, and oil and toss well.

To make the tuna steaks: Dissolve the cornstarch in 1 tablespoon water. In a small saucepan over medium-high heat, combine the orange juice, soy sauce, honey, and red-pepper flakes. Bring the mixture to a boil and cook for 1 minute. Stir in the dissolved cornstarch. Return the mixture to a boil and cook for 1 minute, or until thickened.

In a large nonstick skillet, heat the oil over medium-high heat. Add the tuna steaks and cook for 4 minutes. Turn the tuna and brush with the thickened soy sauce mixture. Cook for 3 to 5 minutes longer, or until the tuna is pink in the center and cooked through. Transfer to a serving platter or dinner plates and brush with any remaining glaze. Serve with the slaw.

Makes 4 servings

Per serving: 300 calories, 43 g protein, 21 g carbohydrates, 5 g fat, 75 mg cholesterol, 660 mg sodium, 2 g dietary fiber
Diet Exchanges: 1 vegetable, 1 bread, 5 meat, ½ fat
Carb Choices: 1

AEGEAN SEAS SHRIMP

Prep time: 20 minutes • Cook time: 12 minutes

1 **pound large shrimp, thawed if frozen, peeled and deveined, rinsed and patted dry**

3 **large cloves garlic, minced**

2 **tablespoons extra-virgin olive oil**

2 **tablespoons lemon juice**

2 **tablespoons chopped fresh oregano or marjoram, or ½ teaspoon dried**

½ **teaspoon sweet paprika**

¼ **teaspoon salt + a pinch**

¼ **teaspoon freshly ground black pepper**

1 **bag (9 ounces) baby spinach**

¼ **cup crumbled feta cheese**

Lemon wedges (optional)

On a rimmed baking sheet, place the shrimp in a mound. Drizzle with 2 minced garlic cloves, 1 tablespoon of the oil, the lemon juice, oregano or marjoram, paprika, the ¼ teaspoon salt, and the pepper. Toss to mix.

Preheat the broiler.

Stir the remaining 1 tablespoon oil and 1 minced garlic clove in a large nonstick skillet over medium heat. Cook, stirring, for 2 minutes, or until the garlic is fragrant. Add the spinach, in batches if necessary, tossing until wilted. Sprinkle with the pinch of salt. Remove from the heat and cover to keep warm.

Broil the shrimp 4" from the heat, turning once, for 3 minutes, or until pink and just firm. Sprinkle with the feta and broil 1 to 2 minutes longer, just until the cheese softens a little (it won't really melt).

Transfer the spinach to a large platter and spoon the shrimp and the pan juices on top. If desired, serve with lemon wedges.

Makes 4 servings

Per serving: 220 calories, 24 g protein, 9 g carbohydrates, 10 g fat, 200 mg cholesterol, 570 mg sodium, 3 g dietary fiber
Diet Exchanges: 1 vegetable, 3 meat, 2 fat
Carb Choices: ½

IT-CAN'T-BE VEGETARIAN MAIN DISHES

FAST SUPER FAST FAST PREP

SPEEDY TAMALE PIE

Photo on page 155.

Prep time: 15 minutes • Cook time: 40 minutes

2   **cans (15 ounces each) salt-free pinto beans, rinsed and drained**

2   **medium zucchini, cut into ¾" chunks**

1   **can (14 ½ ounces) Mexican-style stewed tomatoes**

1   **cup fresh or frozen corn kernels**

1   **cup frozen lima beans**

1   **cup medium-spicy chunky salsa**

2   **teaspoons chili powder**

1   **tube (16–18 ounces) prepared polenta, cut into ½"-thick slices**

1   **cup shredded reduced-fat Cheddar or Monterey Jack cheese**

Preheat the oven to 400°F. Coat a shallow 2 ½-quart baking dish with cooking spray.

In a large soup pot or Dutch oven, combine the beans, zucchini, stewed tomatoes, corn, lima beans, salsa, and chili powder. Bring to a boil. Reduce the heat and simmer, covered, for 10 minutes. Turn into the prepared baking dish. Arrange the polenta on top, overlapping the slices slightly if necessary. Bake for 25 minutes, or until bubbly at the edges. Sprinkle with the cheese and bake for 3 minutes, or until melted. Let stand for 10 minutes before serving.

Makes 6 servings

Per serving: 408 calories, 19 g protein, 77 g carbohydrates, 4 g fat, 5 mg cholesterol, 475 mg sodium, 13 g dietary fiber
Diet Exchanges: 1 ½ vegetable, 4 ½ bread, 2 meat
Carb Choices: 5

BEAN AND VEGGIE BURGERS

Prep time: 25 minutes • Cook time: 35 minutes

BURGERS

¼ cup bulgur

1 small onion, finely chopped

¾ cup shredded zucchini

½ cup shredded carrot

½ cup chopped red bell pepper

1 tablespoon minced garlic

2 cups chopped spinach

1½ teaspoons ground cumin

½ teaspoon salt

4 ounces firm tofu

1 can (15–16 ounces) chickpeas, rinsed and drained

¼ cup ground flaxseed

6 whole wheat buns, split

SAUCE

⅓ cup low-fat plain yogurt

3 tablespoons chopped cilantro

1 scallion, finely chopped

1 jalapeño chile pepper, seeded and minced (wear plastic gloves when handling)

⅛ teaspoon salt

Green leaf lettuce and sliced tomatoes

To make the burgers: Preheat the oven to 400°F. Coat a baking sheet with cooking spray. Prepare the bulgur according to package directions and set aside.

In a large nonstick skillet, over medium heat, combine the onion, zucchini, carrot, bell pepper, and garlic. Cook, stirring frequently, for 8 minutes, or until the vegetables are crisp-tender. Increase the heat to medium-high. Stir in the spinach, cumin, and salt. Cook for 2 minutes, or until the spinach wilts. Cool for 10 minutes.

Pat the tofu dry with paper towels. Crumble the tofu into a large bowl and add the chickpeas. With a potato masher, mash until smooth. Add the vegetable mixture to the bulgur. Stir until well blended. Shape into 6 burgers, 3" in diameter. Coat with the flaxseed. Place on the prepared baking sheet. Bake for 10 minutes. Coat the burgers with cooking spray, and turn over. Bake 15 minutes longer, or until browned.

To make the sauce: In a small bowl, combine the yogurt, cilantro, scallion, chile pepper, and salt. Stir until blended.

Serve each burger on a bun with lettuce, tomato, and yogurt sauce.

Makes 6 servings

Per serving: 260 calories, 13 g protein, 41 g carbohydrates, 7 g fat, 0 mg cholesterol, 620 mg sodium, 9 g dietary fiber
Diet Exchanges: 1 vegetable, 3 bread, $\frac{1}{2}$ meat, $\frac{1}{2}$ fat
Carb Choices: 3

CURRIED TOFU

Photo on page 156.

Prep time: 15 minutes • **Cook time: 50 minutes** • **Stand time: 10 minutes**

1 **cup brown basmati rice**	½ **teaspoon curry powder**
1 **package (14 ounces) firm tofu, drained and cut into ¾" cubes**	4 **cups broccoli florets**
1 **tablespoon canola oil**	1 **cup light coconut milk**
½ **teaspoon salt**	¾ **cup vegetable broth**
1 **large onion, halved and thinly sliced**	1 **cup frozen green peas**
1–2 **tablespoons red curry paste (see note)**	1 **large tomato, cut into ¾" pieces**
	2 **tablespoons lime juice**

Cook the rice according to package directions. Place the tofu between layers of paper towels and let stand for 10 minutes.

Heat the oil in a large nonstick skillet over medium-high heat. Add the tofu and cook, turning once, for 6 to 8 minutes, or until golden brown. Sprinkle with ¼ teaspoon of the salt. With a slotted spoon, remove to a plate.

Add the onion to the skillet and cook, stirring frequently, for 3 to 4 minutes, or until browned. Stir in the curry paste, curry powder, and the remaining ¼ teaspoon salt. Add the broccoli, coconut milk, broth, and peas. Bring to a boil. Reduce the heat to low. Cover and simmer for 3 to 4 minutes, or until the broccoli is crisp-tender. Stir in the tomato, lime juice, and the reserved tofu. Simmer, stirring occasionally, for 2 to 3 minutes, or until the tofu is hot. Serve over the rice.

Note: The heat level of red curry pastes can vary, so start out with 1 tablespoon and then taste.

Makes 6 servings

Per serving: 265 calories, 11 g protein, 37 g carbohydrates, 11 g fat, 0 mg cholesterol, 390 mg sodium, 5 g dietary fiber
Diet Exchanges: 1 ½ vegetable, 2 bread, 1 meat, 1 ½ fat
Carb Choices: 2

BROWN RICE WITH SQUASH AND CHICKPEAS

Prep time: 15 minutes • Cook time: 1 hour 10 minutes

4   teaspoons olive oil

1   medium onion, halved and thinly sliced

3   large cloves garlic, minced

1   tablespoon grated fresh ginger

2 ½   cups water

1   cup brown rice

½   cup lentils

¾   teaspoon salt

1   can (15–19 ounces) chickpeas, rinsed and drained

2   cups frozen cubed butternut squash

2   bunches broccoli rabe, trimmed and cut into 2" pieces

¼–½ teaspoon red-pepper flakes

Heat 2 teaspoons of the oil in a large deep skillet over medium heat. Add the onion. Cook, stirring frequently, for 8 minutes, or until the onion is lightly browned. Add half of the garlic and the ginger. Cook for 1 minute, stirring constantly. Add the water, rice, lentils, and ½ teaspoon of the salt. Bring to a boil. Cover, reduce the heat, and simmer for 30 minutes. Stir in the chickpeas and squash. Cover and cook for 15 to 20 minutes longer, or until the rice is tender.

Meanwhile, bring a large pot of water to a boil. Stir in the broccoli rabe and cook for 2 minutes. Drain, reserving ¼ cup of the cooking water.

In the same pot, heat the remaining 2 teaspoons oil over low heat. Add the red-pepper flakes and the remaining garlic. Cook, stirring constantly, for 1 minute, or until the garlic is sizzling but not brown. Add the broccoli rabe and the remaining ¼ teaspoon salt. Cook, stirring occasionally, for 10 to 12 minutes, or until the broccoli rabe is tender, adding the reserved cooking water if necessary. Serve the rice topped with the broccoli rabe.

Makes 6 servings

Per serving: 312 calories, 13 g protein, 57 g carbohydrates, 5 g fat, 0 mg cholesterol, 490 mg sodium, 11 g dietary fiber
Diet Exchanges: 2 vegetable, 3 bread, 1 meat, ½ fat
Carb Choices: 4

CAJUN RICE WITH RED BEANS AND CORN

Prep time: 15 minutes • Cook time: 1 hour 25 minutes

2 teaspoons canola oil

1 large onion, chopped

1 tablespoon minced garlic

1 tablespoon Cajun or Creole seasoning

2¼ cups water

1 can (15–19 ounces) red or kidney beans, rinsed and drained

1 cup brown rice

1 box (10 ounces) frozen corn

1 green bell pepper, chopped

1 rib celery, chopped

1 can (14 ½ ounces) diced tomatoes

1 scallion, thinly sliced (optional)

   Salt

   Hot-pepper sauce

Heat the oil in a large, deep skillet over medium heat. Add the onion and cook for 5 minutes, or until softened. Stir in the garlic and cook for 1 minute. Stir in the Cajun or Creole seasoning. Remove ½ cup of the onion mixture and set aside. Add the water, beans, and rice. Stir to combine and bring to a boil. Cover, reduce the heat to low, and simmer for 30 minutes. Stir in the corn and cook for 15 to 20 minutes longer, or until the rice is tender.

Meanwhile, in a large saucepan, combine the bell pepper, celery, and the reserved ½ cup onion mixture. Cook over low heat for 10 minutes, or until the vegetables soften. Stir in the tomatoes (with juice) and bring to a boil. Cover, reduce the heat, and simmer for 20 minutes, or until the sauce thickens slightly.

Spoon the rice mixture onto plates and top with the sauce. Sprinkle with the scallion, if using. Add the salt to taste. Serve with the hot-pepper sauce on the side.

Makes 6 servings

Per serving: 250 calories, 8 g protein, 50 g carbohydrates, 3 g fat, 0 mg cholesterol, 210 mg sodium, 8 g dietary fiber
Diet Exchanges: 1 vegetable, 3 bread, ½ fat
Carb Choices: 3

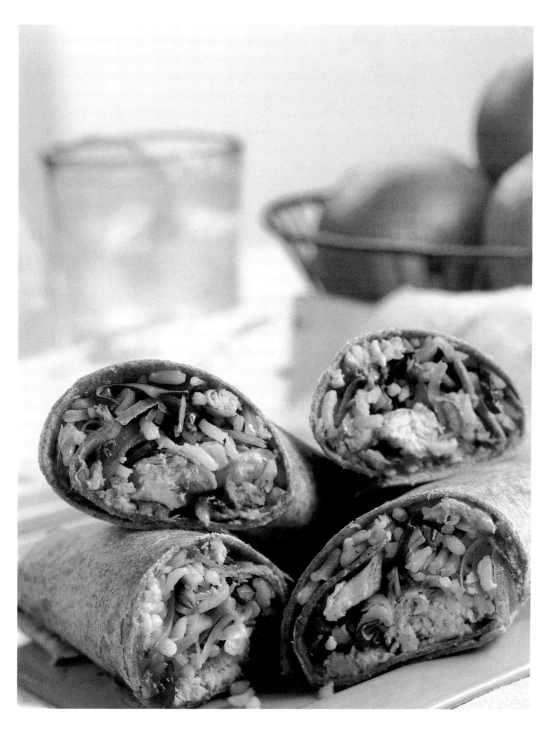

PEKING CHICKEN WRAPS

Recipe on page 133

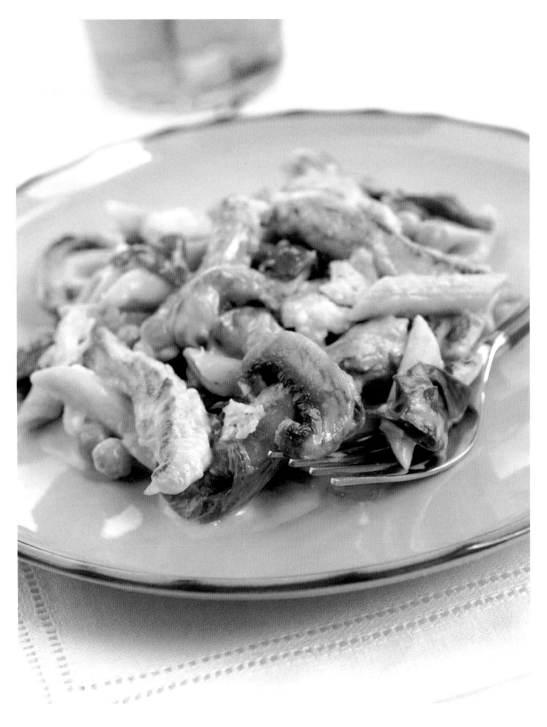

SKILLET TURKEY TETRAZZINI

Recipe on page 139

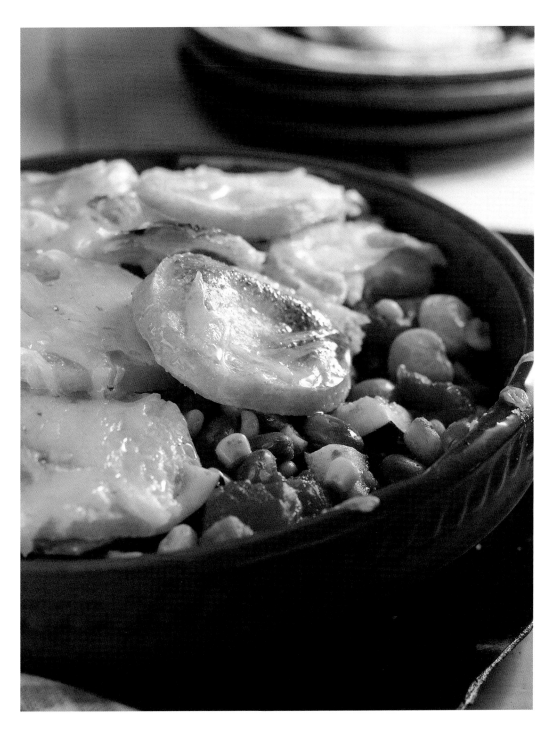

SPEEDY TAMALE PIE

Recipes on pages 147

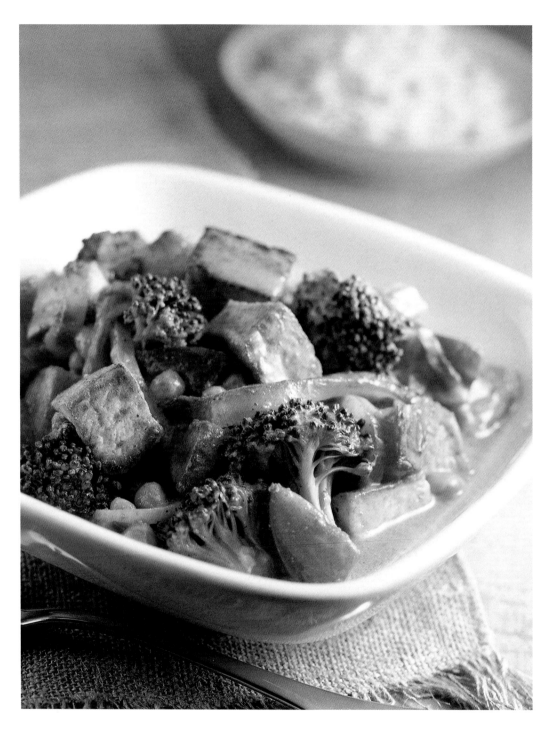

CURRIED TOFU

Recipe on page 150

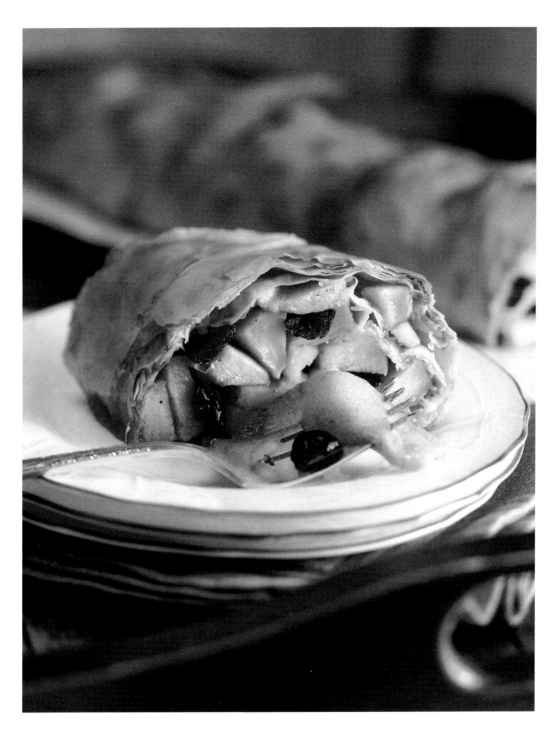

ROASTED APPLE-CRANBERRY STRUDEL

Recipe on page 172

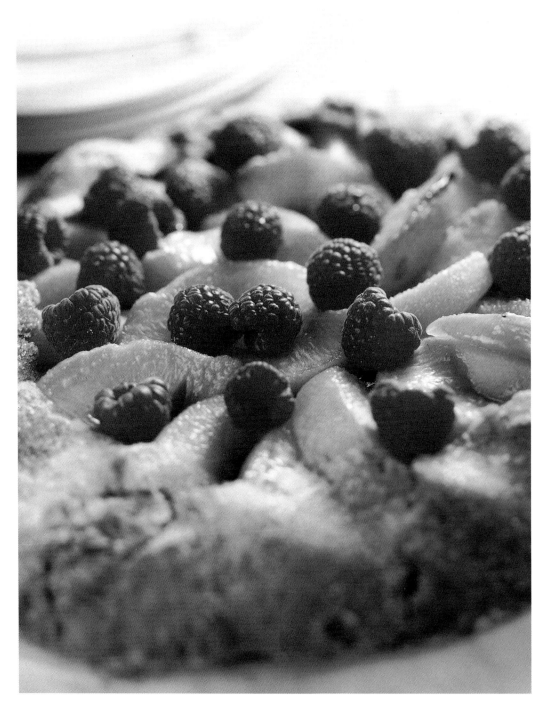

PEACH AND RASPBERRY CROSTATA

Recipe on page 176

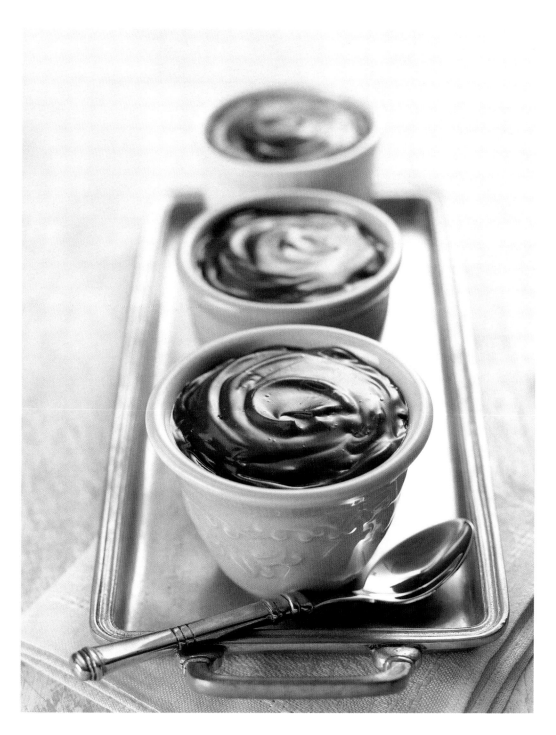

DARK CHOCOLATE PUDDING

Recipe on page 179

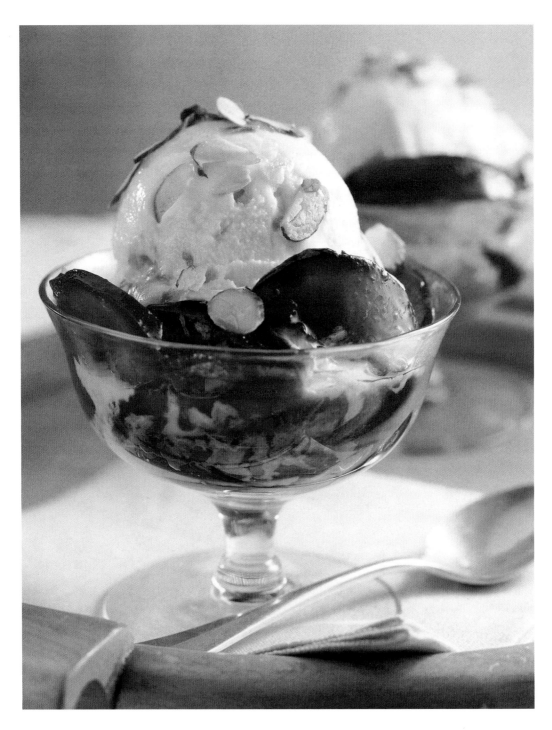

GINGER FROZEN YOGURT WITH SWEET PLUM SAUCE

Recipe on page 181

STUFFED PORTOBELLOS

Prep time: 20 minutes • Cook time: 35 minutes

1 cup brown rice

2 teaspoons olive oil

1 small onion, chopped

4 cups sliced escarole or Swiss chard

2 large cloves garlic, minced

½ cup rinsed and chopped roasted red peppers

4 large portobello mushrooms (4 ½"–5" diameter), stems discarded (see note)

½ cup prepared hummus, preferably basil flavored

3 plum tomatoes, sliced

¼ cup walnuts, chopped

¼ cup grated Parmesan cheese

Preheat the oven to 400°F.

Cook the rice according to package directions.

Meanwhile, heat the oil in a medium skillet over medium-low heat. Add the onion and cook, stirring occasionally, for 5 minutes, or until softened. Add the escarole or Swiss chard and the garlic. Cook, stirring occasionally, for 5 minutes, or until wilted. Remove from the heat and stir in the rice and peppers.

Place the mushrooms gill side up on a baking sheet with sides. Spread the hummus on the mushrooms and spoon on the rice mixture, spreading it to the edges. Arrange the tomato slices on top and sprinkle with the walnuts and cheese. Bake for 25 to 30 minutes, or until the mushrooms are tender. Let stand for 10 minutes before serving.

Note: To prevent the mushrooms from being waterlogged, remove any sand or dirt with a brush and wipe with damp paper towels instead of rinsing with water.

Makes 4 servings

Per serving: 260 calories, 10 g protein, 30 g carbohydrates, 12 g fat, 5 mg cholesterol, 250 mg sodium, 7 g dietary fiber
Diet Exchanges: 3 vegetable, 1 bread, 1 meat, 2 fat
Carb Choices: 2

ITALIAN VEGETABLE STIR-FRY OVER POLENTA

Prep time: 20 minutes • Cook time: 35 minutes

POLENTA

4 cups water

¼ teaspoon salt

1 cup yellow cornmeal

½ cup grated Parmesan cheese

STIR-FRY

1 tablespoon olive oil

1 small red onion, thinly sliced

1 red bell pepper, thinly sliced

1 small fennel bulb, trimmed, quartered, cored, and thinly sliced

1 large zucchini, halved lengthwise and thinly sliced

1 can (15–19 ounces) chickpeas, rinsed and drained

1 tablespoon minced garlic

¼ teaspoon red-pepper flakes

¼ teaspoon salt

2 large tomatoes, coarsely chopped

¼ cup chopped fresh basil

To make the polenta: In a large saucepan, bring the water and salt to a boil. Slowly whisk in the cornmeal. Reduce the heat to low. Cover and simmer, stirring frequently, for 30 to 35 minutes, or until the polenta thickens. Stir in the cheese. Cover and keep warm.

To make the stir-fry: Heat the oil in a large nonstick skillet over medium-high heat. Add the onion, bell pepper, and fennel. Cook, stirring frequently, for 2 to 3 minutes, or until the vegetables begin to soften. Add the zucchini, chickpeas, garlic, red-pepper flakes, and salt. Cook, stirring constantly, for 2 to 3 minutes, or until the vegetables are crisp-tender. Add the tomatoes. Cook, stirring frequently, for 1 minute, or until the tomatoes soften. Stir in the basil. Serve over the polenta.

Makes 6 servings

Per serving: 246 calories, 10 g protein, 38 g carbohydrates, 7 g fat, 5 mg cholesterol, 580 mg sodium, 7 g dietary fiber
Diet Exchanges: 1 ½ vegetable, 2 bread, ½ meat, 1 fat
Carb Choices: 3

CHUNKY VEGETABLE SHEPHERD'S PIE

Prep time: 30 minutes • Cook time: 1 hour 10 minutes

3 pounds sweet potatoes, peeled and cut into large chunks

1 tablespoon olive oil

1 large onion, coarsely chopped

3 medium carrots, sliced

1 large rib celery, sliced

½ pound cremini mushrooms, halved

1 tablespoon minced garlic

1 teaspoon seasoning blend, such as Mrs. Dash original

1 can (15–19 ounces) cannellini beans, rinsed and drained

1 box (9 ounces) frozen Italian green beans

1 can (14 ounces) vegetable broth

3 tablespoons whole grain pastry flour

4 plum tomatoes, cut into ¾" pieces

In a soup pot or Dutch oven, cover the potatoes with cold water. Bring to a boil. Cover, reduce the heat, and simmer for 15 to 20 minutes, or until tender. Drain in a colander and set aside.

Preheat the oven to 375°F.

In the same pot, heat the oil over medium heat. Add the onion, carrots, and celery. Cook, stirring occasionally, for 5 minutes, or until the onion softens. Stir in the mushrooms, garlic, and seasoning blend. Cook, stirring frequently, for 5 minutes, or until the mushrooms soften. Add the cannellini, green beans, and broth. Bring to a boil. In a small bowl, whisk ½ cup cold water and the flour until smooth. Stir into the vegetables. Reduce the heat and simmer for 3 minutes. Stir in the tomatoes. Pour the vegetable mixture into a 13" × 9" baking dish.

In the same pot, mash the sweet potatoes. Spoon the potatoes around the edge of the baking dish. Bake for 35 minutes, or until bubbly in the center. Let stand for 5 minutes before serving.

Makes 8 servings

Per serving: 299 calories, 10 g protein, 63 g carbohydrates, 2 g fat, 0 mg cholesterol, 460 mg sodium, 11 g dietary fiber
Diet Exchanges: 2 vegetable, 3 ½ bread
Carb Choices: 4

TO-DIE-FOR DESSERTS

■ FAST   ■ SUPER FAST   ■ FAST PREP

CHOCOLATE ALMOND MERINGUE COOKIES

Prep time: 20 minutes • Cook time: 2 hours

½ cup blanched almonds

5 tablespoons sugar

3 large egg whites, at room temperature

¼ teaspoon cream of tartar

2 tablespoons unsweetened cocoa powder

¼ cup raspberry or strawberry all-fruit preserves

Preheat the oven to 250°F. Line a baking sheet with parchment paper or foil.

Place the almonds and 2 tablespoons of the sugar in a food processor. Process until finely ground.

Place the egg whites and cream of tartar in a large bowl. Using an electric mixer on high speed, beat until frothy. Gradually add the remaining 3 tablespoons sugar and beat until stiff, glossy peaks form. Gently fold in the cocoa and ground almonds.

Spoon the meringue into 1½" mounds on the prepared baking sheet. Using the back of a spoon, depress the centers and build up the sides of each meringue to form a shallow cup.

Bake for 1 hour. Turn off the oven and allow the meringues to stand with the oven door closed for 1 hour. Remove from the sheet and place onto a rack to cool completely.

Store in an airtight container. To serve, fill each meringue with ¼ teaspoon of the preserves.

Makes 16

Per cookie: 61 calories, 2 g protein, 9 g carbohydrates, 2 g fat, 0 mg cholesterol, 10 mg sodium, 1 g dietary fiber
Diet Exchanges: ½ bread, ½ fat
Carb Choice: 1

CRUNCHY PEANUT SQUARES

Prep time: 5 minutes • Cook time: 3 minutes

1 **tablespoon butter**	3 **cups plain air-popped popcorn**
⅓ **cup honey**	2 **cups crisp rice cereal**
¼ **cup packed brown sugar**	2 **cups oat circle cereal**
⅓ **cup natural peanut butter**	⅓ **cup unsalted peanuts, chopped**
1 **teaspoon vanilla extract**	⅓ **cup chocolate chips (optional)**

Line a 13" × 9" × 2" baking pan with foil, extending the foil at the ends. Coat the foil with cooking spray.

In a large nonstick saucepan, melt the butter, honey, and brown sugar over low heat, stirring frequently. Remove the saucepan from the heat. Add the peanut butter and vanilla. Return the saucepan to the heat and cook, stirring constantly, for 2 minutes, until the mixture is well blended and melts.

Remove the pan from the heat and add the popcorn, rice and oat cereals, and peanuts. Stir until evenly coated with the peanut butter mixture. Turn into the prepared pan. Spray hands with cooking spray and press the mixture firmly into the pan. Sprinkle with chocolate chips, if using. Cool completely on a rack.

Remove from the pan using the foil. Discard the foil. Cut into squares to serve.

Makes 24

Per square: 82 calories, 2 g protein, 12 g carbohydrates, 3 g fat, 0 mg cholesterol, 65 mg sodium, 1 g dietary fiber
Diet Exchanges: ½ bread, ½ fat
Carb Choices: 1

DOUBLE CHERRY–CORNMEAL TEA BREAD

Prep time: 20 minutes • Cook time: 55 minutes • Stand time: 10 minutes

3 tablespoons dried cherries	⅓ cup plain low-fat yogurt
1 ⅓ cups whole grain pastry flour	¼ cup unsweetened applesauce
⅔ cup yellow cornmeal	2 tablespoons butter, melted
1 teaspoon baking powder	1 egg
½ teaspoon baking soda	1 tablespoon grated orange or lemon peel
¼ teaspoon salt	1 cup fresh cherries, pitted and quartered
⅔ cup sugar	

Preheat the oven to 350°F. Coat an 8 ½" × 4 ½" loaf pan with cooking spray. In a small dish, combine the dried cherries with enough hot water to cover. Let stand for 10 minutes, or until softened.

Meanwhile, in a medium bowl, whisk together the flour, cornmeal, baking powder, baking soda, and salt until blended. In a medium bowl, whisk together the sugar, yogurt, applesauce, butter, egg, and orange or lemon peel until well blended. Drain the dried cherries well and coarsely chop. Stir the fresh and dried cherries into the yogurt mixture. Add the flour mixture in 2 additions, stirring just until combined. Scrape the batter into the prepared pan.

Bake for 55 minutes, or until a wooden pick inserted into the center comes out clean. Cool in the pan on a rack for 10 minutes. Turn out onto the rack and cool completely.

Makes 12 servings

Per serving: 141 calories, 3 g protein, 25 g carbohydrates, 3 g fat, 25 mg cholesterol, 180 mg sodium, 2 g dietary fiber
Diet Exchanges: 1 ½ bread, ½ fat
Carb Choices: 2

OATMEAL-DATE BARS

Prep time: 30 minutes • **Cook time: 35 minutes**

FILLING

1 cup cinnamon applesauce, sweetened with apple juice concentrate

1 cup chopped dates

½ teaspoon pumpkin pie spice

1 teaspoon vanilla extract

CRUST

1 cup whole grain pastry flour

1 cup old-fashioned rolled oats

½ teaspoon baking powder

½ teaspoon baking soda

½ teaspoon salt

⅔ cup packed brown sugar

3 tablespoons butter, at room temperature

3 tablespoons reduced-fat sour cream

Preheat the oven to 375°F. Line a 10 ½" × 7" baking dish with foil and coat with cooking spray.

To make the filling: In a small nonstick saucepan, combine the applesauce, dates, and pumpkin pie spice. Bring to a bare simmer and cook 10 minutes, or until thickened, stirring and mashing occasionally with a heatproof spatula. Stir the vanilla into the filling until blended and set the filling aside to cool while preparing the crust.

To make the crust: In a medium bowl, whisk together the flour, oats, baking powder, baking soda, and salt. Place the mixture on a sheet of waxed paper. In the same bowl, beat the sugar, butter, and sour cream with an electric mixer on high speed for 1 minute. Stir in the oat mixture with a wooden spoon until combined.

Set a sheet of plastic wrap on a small baking sheet. Remove 1 cup of the dough and crumble it onto the plastic wrap. Cover loosely with the plastic and freeze while assembling the bars. Drop the remaining dough by spoonfuls into the prepared baking dish. Cover with a sheet of plastic wrap coated with cooking spray and press the dough into an even layer. Remove the wrap.

Drop the filling by spoonfuls over the dough and spread in an even layer. Crumble the chilled dough evenly over the filling.

Bake for 25 minutes, or until golden brown. Cool completely in the pan on a rack. Remove from the pan and gently remove the foil. Cut into 18 squares, cutting in thirds lengthwise and sixths crosswise. Store airtight for up to 1 week, or freeze for up to 2 months.

Makes 18

Per bar: 96 calories, 2 g protein, 18 g carbohydrates, 3 g fat, 5 mg cholesterol, 135 mg sodium, 2 g dietary fiber
Diet Exchanges: 1 fruit, ½ bread, ½ fat
Carb Choices: 1

PEANUT BUTTER BUNDT CAKE

Prep time: 25 minutes • **Cook time: 55 minutes**

CAKE

1 ½ cups whole grain pastry flour

1 cup cake flour

2 teaspoons baking powder

½ teaspoon baking soda

½ teaspoon salt

½ cup reduced-fat peanut butter

½ cup butter, at room temperature

1 cup sugar

2 egg whites

1 tablespoon vanilla extract

⅓ cup mini chocolate chips

1 ½ cups low-fat buttermilk

GLAZE

1 tablespoon unsweetened cocoa powder

2 tablespoons peanut butter

1 ½–2 tablespoons water

½ teaspoon vanilla extract

½ cup confectioners' sugar

Pinch of salt

To make the cake: Preheat the oven to 350°F. Coat a 10" Bundt pan with cooking spray.

In a medium bowl, whisk together the whole grain and cake flours, baking powder, baking soda, and salt. In another medium bowl with an electric mixer at medium speed, beat together the peanut butter and butter for 1 minute, or until creamy. Add the sugar, egg whites, and vanilla and beat for 2 minutes, or until light and fluffy. Beat in the chocolate chips on low speed, just until combined.

With the mixer set on the lowest speed, alternately add the flour mixture and the buttermilk in 3 additions, beginning and ending with the flour mixture. Scrape the batter into the prepared pan and spread level.

Bake for 55 to 60 minutes, or until a wooden pick inserted into the center comes out clean and the cake begins to pull away from the sides of the pan. Cool in the pan on a rack for 10 minutes. Loosen the sides with a spatula and invert onto a serving plate. Slip strips of waxed paper under the edges of the cake, for glazing.

To make the glaze: Meanwhile, in a small bowl, stir together the cocoa, peanut butter, water, and vanilla until blended. Stir in the confectioners' sugar and salt until smooth. Drizzle the glaze over the cake using a spoon. Set aside until the glaze is firm. Remove the waxed paper strips.

Makes 16 servings

Per serving: 270 calories, 6 g protein, 37 g carbohydrates, 12 g fat, 15 mg cholesterol, 290 mg sodium, 2 g dietary fiber
Diet Exchanges: 2 $\frac{1}{2}$ bread, $\frac{1}{2}$ meat, 3 fat
Carb Choices: 3

ROASTED APPLE-CRANBERRY STRUDEL

Photo on page 157.

Prep time: 35 minutes • Cook time: 32 minutes • Stand time: 10 minutes

4 large Granny Smith apples (2 $\frac{1}{4}$ pounds), peeled, cored, and thinly sliced

$\frac{1}{3}$ cup dried cranberries

1 tablespoon brandy or water

$\frac{1}{2}$ teaspoon pumpkin pie spice or ground nutmeg

$\frac{1}{3}$ cup + 1 $\frac{1}{2}$ tablespoons packed brown sugar

$\frac{3}{4}$ teaspoon ground cinnamon

5 sheets phyllo dough (17" $\times$ 12")

3 tablespoons butter, melted

Preheat the oven to 400°F. Line 2 large baking sheets with foil and coat with cooking spray.

Spread the apple slices in an even layer on one of the baking sheets. Bake for 12 minutes, or until tender, turning them over with a fork or spatula halfway through the cooking (for microwave directions, see note). Meanwhile, in a small microwaveable bowl, combine the cranberries and brandy or water. Cover loosely with plastic wrap and microwave on high for 40 seconds, or until the liquid just begins to simmer. Let stand for at least 10 minutes.

Spoon the apples into a medium bowl (you should have about 2 $\frac{1}{2}$ cups). Stir in the pie spice or nutmeg, the $\frac{1}{3}$ cup sugar, $\frac{1}{2}$ teaspoon of the cinnamon, and the cranberries. Set aside to cool.

In a small dish, stir together the 1 $\frac{1}{2}$ tablespoons sugar and the remaining $\frac{1}{4}$ teaspoon cinnamon. Lay 1 sheet of phyllo on a sheet of waxed paper and lightly brush with the butter. Sprinkle evenly with about one-quarter of the cinnamon sugar. Repeat with the remaining phyllo, butter, and cinnamon sugar, coating the last phyllo with butter only, layering the phyllo sheets on top of each other.

Mound the apple mixture down the long side of the phyllo stack, leaving a 2" border on the long side and the ends. Loosely roll up the strudel, using the waxed paper as a guide. Tuck in the ends and transfer to the prepared baking sheet. Brush the top of the strudel with the remaining butter. Using a serrated knife, divide the strudel into 8 equal portions by cutting lightly through the top of the strudel (just to the filling), on the diagonal. Do not cut all the way through.

Bake for 20 to 25 minutes, or just until golden brown. Cool in the pan on a rack for at least 10 minutes. Slide the strudel onto a board and cut along the scored marks. Serve warm.

Note: To "bake" apples in the microwave, place them in a microwaveable glass bowl and microwave on high power for 2 to 3 minutes, stirring once. Apples should be tender enough to pierce with fork.

Makes 8 servings

Per serving: 188 calories, 1 g protein, 35 g carbohydrates, 5 g fat, 10 mg cholesterol, 105 mg sodium, 4 g dietary fiber
Diet Exchanges: 1 fruit, 1 bread, 1 fat
Carb Choices: 2

BLUEBERRY-GINGER CRUMB PIE

Prep time: 10 minutes • Cook time: 18 minutes

CRUST

1 **cup gingersnap cookies (about 7 ounces)**   2 **tablespoons butter, melted**

1 ½ **tablespoons brown sugar**

FILLING

5–6 **cups fresh or frozen and thawed blueberries**   ¼ **cup water**

4 **tablespoons cornstarch**   ½ **cup granulated sugar**

To make the crust: Preheat the oven to 325°F. Place the gingersnaps in a food processor and process until the crumbs are fine. Add the brown sugar and butter and pulse the processor until the mixture is just combined.

Press into a 9" pie plate and bake for 8 to 10 minutes. Let cool.

To make the filling: Place the blueberries, cornstarch, and water in a medium saucepan. Bring to a simmer over medium heat until slightly thickened. Add the granulated sugar and heat on low for 10 to 12 minutes, until the sugar is dissolved. Remove from the heat and cool slightly. Pour the filling into the prepared crust. Cool completely before cutting.

Makes 8 servings

Per serving: 220 calories, 2 g protein, 45 g carbohydrates, 5 g fat, 10 mg cholesterol, 135 mg sodium, 3 g dietary fiber
Diet Exchanges: 1 fruit, 2 ½ bread, 1 ½ fat
Carb Choices: 4

STRAWBERRY-RHUBARB CRISP

Prep time: 25 minutes • Cook time: 35 minutes • Stand time: 20 minutes

2 pints strawberries, hulled and quartered lengthwise

2 cups fresh or frozen and thawed rhubarb (cut into 1/2" pieces)

1–2 tablespoons quick-cooking tapioca, or 1/2–1 tablespoon cornstarch (see note)

1/4 teaspoon ground ginger

3/4 cup sugar

1 teaspoon ground cinnamon

1/3 cup whole grain pastry flour

Pinch of salt

2 tablespoons butter

1/2 cup old-fashioned rolled oats

1 1/2 tablespoons honey

In a 2-quart baking dish, combine the strawberries, rhubarb, tapioca or cornstarch, ginger, 1/2 cup of the sugar, and 1/4 teaspoon of the cinnamon. Spread the fruit mixture level, and let stand for 20 minutes.

Meanwhile, preheat the oven to 400°F. In a medium bowl, stir together the flour, salt, and the remaining 1/4 cup sugar, and 3/4 teaspoon cinnamon. Cut in the butter until the mixture is the texture of fine meal. Stir in the oats until combined. Drizzle the honey on top and stir until the mixture is crumbly. Sprinkle over the fruit in an even layer.

Bake for 35 to 40 minutes, or until the fruit is bubbly and the topping is golden brown. Serve warm or at room temperature.

Note: If the berries are not very juicy, use the minimum amount of cornstarch suggested in the recipe.

Makes 6 servings

Per serving: 232 calories, 3 g protein, 47 g carbohydrates, 5 g fat, 10 mg cholesterol, 0 mg sodium, 5 g dietary fiber
Diet Exchanges: 1 fruit, 2 bread, 1 fat
Carb Choices: 3

PEACH AND RASPBERRY CROSTATA

Photo on page 158.

Prep time: 40 minutes • Cook time: 45 minutes • Stand time: 30 minutes

CRUST

1½ cups whole grain pastry flour

¼ teaspoon salt

¼ cup vegetable shortening

2 ounces reduced-fat cream cheese

2 teaspoons lemon juice

4–5 tablespoons ice water

TOPPING

3 tablespoons shredded bran cereal

1 tablespoon whole grain pastry flour

¼ teaspoon ground cinnamon

6 tablespoons sugar

1¾ pounds fresh peaches, peeled and pitted (see note)

1 cup fresh raspberries

To make the crust: In a large bowl, combine the flour and salt. Cut in the shortening and cream cheese until the mixture resembles coarse crumbs. In a cup, stir the lemon juice together with 2 tablespoons of the water. Drizzle over the crumb mixture and mix until moistened. Mix in the remaining water 1 tablespoon at a time, until the texture resembles cottage cheese and it can be pressed into a firm ball.

Press the dough into a 6" disk. Wrap in plastic wrap and refrigerate at least 30 minutes before using.

Place a wide sheet of foil onto a large baking sheet and coat with cooking spray. Fold the edges of the foil up ½" to form a rim. Roll the dough out between sheets of lightly floured waxed paper to a 13" circle. Place onto the prepared baking sheet, cover with plastic wrap, and refrigerate until using.

To make the topping: Preheat the oven to 400°F.

In a food processor or blender, combine the cereal, flour, cinnamon, and 4 tablespoons of the sugar. Process until the cereal is finely ground. Sprinkle the cereal mixture over the pastry, leaving a 2" border. Arrange the peaches over the cereal mixture. Fold the pastry border over the fruit. Sprinkle the remaining 2 tablespoons of sugar over the fruit and the pastry edge.

Bake for 45 to 50 minutes, or until the crust is golden brown and juices are bubbly. Cool in the pan on a rack. Sprinkle on the raspberries.

Note: To substitute frozen peaches, use 1 ½ pounds dry-packed sliced peaches, thawing in a single layer on paper towels to absorb excess liquid.

Makes 10 servings

Per serving: 181 calories, 3 g protein, 30 g carbohydrates, 6 g fat, 5 mg cholesterol, 90 mg sodium, 4 g dietary fiber
Diet Exchanges: 1 fruit, 1 bread, 1 fat
Carb Choices: 2

ROASTED PEARS WITH ORANGE-CARAMEL SAUCE

Prep time: 20 minutes • Cook time: 50 minutes

2 **tablespoons hazelnuts, chopped**	¼ **cup orange juice, at room temperature**
1 **tablespoon butter**	4 **dried figs, stemmed and chopped**
⅓ **cup sugar**	1 **tablespoon orange liqueur (optional)**
4 **ripe pears, halved and cored**	

Place the hazelnuts in a dry skillet and cook over medium heat for 4 minutes, or until fragrant. Be sure to stir the nuts frequently to prevent burning. Set aside.

Preheat the oven to 400°F. Spread the butter in the bottom of a 13" × 9" × 2" baking dish. Sprinkle with 2 tablespoons of the sugar. Place the pear halves cut side down in the prepared baking dish. Bake for 35 to 40 minutes, or until the pears are tender when pierced with the tip of a knife.

Meanwhile, place the remaining sugar in a small saucepan. Cook over medium-high heat, swirling the pan frequently, for 5 minutes, until the sugar melts and turns amber in color. Remove the pan from the heat and slowly pour in the orange juice to avoid sputtering hot liquid. Return the pan to medium-low heat. Cook the sauce, stirring constantly, for 5 minutes, until the sauce thickens slightly. Stir in the figs and liqueur, if using. Set the sauce aside.

Remove the pears from the baking dish to serving plates. Add any juices remaining in the baking dish to the sauce.

Serve the pears warm or at room temperature. Spoon the sauce over the pears and sprinkle with the hazelnuts. If the sauce thickens after sitting, rewarm it over low heat.

Makes 4 servings

Per serving: 260 calories, 2 g protein, 54 g carbohydrates, 6 g fat, 10 mg cholesterol, 20 mg sodium, 6 g dietary fiber
Diet Exchanges: 2 ½ fruit, 1 ½ bread, 1 fat
Carb Choices: 4

DARK CHOCOLATE PUDDING

Photo on page 159.

FAST

Prep time: 10 minutes • Cook time: 12 minutes • Chill: 2 hours

¼ cup sugar

¼ cup malted milk powder

3 tablespoons unsweetened cocoa powder

2 tablespoons cornstarch

1 teaspoon instant coffee powder

2 cups 1% milk

1 ounce unsweetened chocolate, finely chopped

1 teaspoon vanilla extract

In a medium saucepan, whisk together the sugar, malted milk powder, cocoa, cornstarch, and coffee powder until blended. Gradually whisk in the milk.

Cook over medium heat, stirring constantly, for 10 minutes until the pudding thickens and comes to a boil. Reduce the heat to low and add the chocolate. Cook, stirring constantly, for 1 minute, until the chocolate melts. Remove from the heat and stir in the vanilla. Pour the pudding into 4 custard cups. Cover with plastic wrap and refrigerate until cold, at least 2 hours.

Note: A heatproof rubber spatula works well for stirring the pudding to prevent it from scorching on the bottom.

Makes 4 servings

Per serving: 250 calories, 8 g protein, 46 g carbohydrates, 6 g fat, 5 mg cholesterol, 125 mg sodium, 4 g dietary fiber
Diet Exchanges: ½ milk, 3 bread, ½ fat
Carb Choices: 3

BROWN RICE PUDDING

Prep time: 20 minutes • **Cook time: 1 hour 20 minutes** • **Chill time: 4 hours or overnight**

1 ¼ cups water

1 tablespoon grated lemon peel

¼ teaspoon salt

½ cup brown rice

3 cups 2% milk

1 tablespoon vanilla extract

3 tablespoons packed brown sugar

Chopped mango or papaya (optional)

¼ cup shredded sweetened coconut (optional)

In a large saucepan, combine the water, 1 ½ teaspoons of the lemon peel, and the salt. Bring to a boil and add the rice. Reduce the heat and simmer, covered, for 40 minutes, or until the rice is tender and most of the water is absorbed.

Stir in the milk, vanilla, sugar, and the remaining lemon peel. Bring to a boil. Reduce the heat to low and simmer for 40 to 45 minutes, stirring frequently to prevent sticking, especially toward the end of the cooking time, until the pudding thickens and the rice is very tender. (It will thicken more on standing.) Pour the pudding into a bowl and let cool to room temperature, stirring occasionally. Cover with plastic wrap and refrigerate 4 hours (or overnight) until chilled.

To serve, spoon the pudding into 6 individual serving dishes. Top with the mango or papaya, if using, and coconut, if using.

Makes 6 servings

Per serving: 141 calories, 5 g protein, 25 g carbohydrates, 2 g fat, 5 mg cholesterol, 160 mg sodium, 1 g dietary fiber
Diet Exchanges: ½ milk, 1 ½ bread
Carb Choices: 2

GINGER FROZEN YOGURT WITH SWEET PLUM SAUCE

Photo on page 160.

Prep time: 10 minutes • Cook time: 35 minutes

¼ cup sliced almonds

1 pint fat-free vanilla frozen yogurt, slightly softened

2–4 tablespoons finely chopped crystallized ginger

1 pound ripe plums (4 large), pitted and sliced

3 tablespoons sugar-free grape jam

1 tablespoon sugar

Preheat the oven to 300°F. Spread the almonds on a baking sheet. Bake for 10 minutes, or until lightly toasted. Let cool, then coarsely chop the almonds.

In a large bowl, combine the frozen yogurt and ginger. Quickly stir to combine. Return the yogurt to the freezer.

In a medium saucepan, combine the plums, jam, and sugar. Bring to a simmer over medium heat. Reduce the heat to low, cover, and simmer for 12 minutes, until the plums soften and break down. Uncover and simmer for 5 minutes, until the sauce thickens slightly. Pour the sauce into a bowl and let cool. Cover with plastic wrap and refrigerate until cold.

To serve, spoon the sauce into 4 individual serving dishes. Top with scoops of the frozen yogurt and sprinkle with the almonds.

Makes 4 servings

Per serving: 200 calories, 6 g protein, 39 g carbohydrates, 4 g fat, 0 mg cholesterol, 80 mg sodium, 2 g dietary fiber
Diet Exchanges: 1 fruit, 2 ½ bread, 1 fat
Carb Choices: 4

LEMON PUDDING CAKE

Prep time: 25 minutes • Cook time: 40 minutes

½ cup sugar

3 tablespoons whole grain pastry flour

⅛ teaspoon ground nutmeg

1 cup 1% milk or unsweetened light soymilk

¼ cup lemon juice

2 tablespoons butter, melted

1 egg yolk

1 ½ teaspoons grated lemon peel

2 large egg whites

⅛ teaspoon salt

Preheat the oven to 350°F. Set a 1-quart soufflé or baking dish in a small roasting pan.

In a medium bowl, combine the sugar, flour, and nutmeg. Make a well in the center. Add the milk or soymilk, lemon juice, butter, egg yolk, and lemon peel. Mix by hand until blended.

With an electric mixer on medium-high speed, beat the egg whites and salt in a medium bowl until soft peaks form. Spoon the whites into the batter and fold together until smooth. (The batter will be thin.) Pour into the soufflé or baking dish. Add boiling water to the roasting pan to come halfway up the side of the dish.

Bake for 40 minutes, or until the top is golden and a pudding has formed underneath. (Cut a small slit in the center to ensure that the cake layer is done.) Remove the baking dish to a rack and cool for 15 minutes. Serve warm or at room temperature.

Makes 4 servings

Per serving: 214 calories, 5 g protein, 33 g carbohydrates, 8 g fat, 70 mg cholesterol, 210 mg sodium, 1 g dietary fiber
Diet Exchanges: 2 bread, 1 ½ fat
Carb Choices: 2

INDEX